"The history of the healing virtues of plants dates back to the dawn of man's existence on earth. The great interest in herbs today is evidenced not only because they are being used more skillfully for the purpose of healing, but by the fact that many people are choosing herbs over the risk and side-effects that accompany so many modern pharmaceuticals. This is a wonderfully informative book providing step by step instructions on how to use tea tree oil as a valid alternative and adjunct to orthodox pharmacy.

Echoing the words of medicine's Hippocratic Oath, primum non nocere, West shares with her readers a therapy which is safe, natural, effective, and without harmful side-effects. It is truly an essential addition to anyone's health library."

MARIA-CHELARU-WILLIAMS DVM
Alternative Medical Approach
For Animals Clinic

"I have been successfully using tea tree oil for the past year or so. I find (this book) extremely informative and useful.It will be of great value to anyone wanting to use an alternative method to traditional veterinarian products for treating animals."

ANGELA LANGDON-NEILSON
Editor Walking Horse News/Steppin' Out
Publication

"A comprehensive guide to the uses of tea tree oil for animals. It offers easy to use techniques to improve the health of our animals companions. From horses to pot bellied pigs, Cheyanne West offers a wide range of uses for tea tree oil. Easy to use and clearly written, this is a book for every one interested in natural animal health care."

KATRINA PRULL -Chamisa Ridge

Australian Tea Tree Oil

First Aid for Animals

Cheyanne West

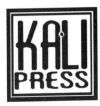

The treatments offered here in this book are related to you through experience. Tea tree oil is not a substitute to good veterinarian care; however, it does offer an alternative to using harsh chemicals or other abrasive treatments. Not all animals react the same to tea tree oil or its treatment. If any condition persists, consult with your veterinarian.

First Published in 1998 by :
Kali Press
Box 2169
Pagosa Springs, CO 81147-2169

Publisher's Cataloging-in-Publication Data:
(Provided by Quality Books, Inc.)
West, Cheyanne.
    Australian tea tree oil: first aid for animals/
Cheyanne West; [editing and illustrations by
Penelope Greenwell]. --1st ed.
    p.cm.
    Includes bibliographical references and index
    Preassigned LCCN: 98-66189.
    ISBN: 0-9628882-7-3

    1. First Aid for animals 2. Melaleuca alternifolia oil
    3. Alternative veterinary medicine. I. Title.

SF914.3.W47 1988   636.089
                        QBI98-883

10 9 8 7 6 5 4 3 2 1

Editing: C. Gerlach, Morgan Caldwell
Cover design, interior design and illustrations:
Penelope Greenwell, Pentangle Press
Cover photograph of Tea Trees:
Maincamp NSW, Australia
Illustration of Goat - page 86:
Sue Tinkle

Dedication

To Richard Running Deer;
who's love and support
keeps me looking forward.
And to all those who love their animals
enough to treat them with natural therapies.

Author's Acknowledgements

My heartfelt thanks to my special friend, Cynthia Olsen, whose encouragement made this book possible. To Char Chambers, who introduced me to Tea Tree Oil in the mid 1980's. To Penny Greenwell who made this book come alive with her creative talents. And finally, to all the creatures I have worked with throughout the years and their owners who thought enough of their animals to seek a better alternative.

TABLE OF CONTENTS

Foreword

$\mathcal{I}$ love animals, my four-legged ones, that is. When I was growing up, my mother never permitted animals to live with us. She couldn't cope with the puppy training, the messes, shedding, and anything else that was associated with an animal. Once my dad brought home a cocker spaniel, to my mother's horror. She banned the puppy to the basement and told my father the puppy had to be gone by the next morning.

My aunt called one day and announced to my mother that they were getting a boxer puppy and wanted me to come along with them. I remember sitting in the back seat of their car with the puppy in a little box beside me. My aunt said, "why don't you give the puppy a name." I was very pleased. I named the dog Chips. From that day on, Chips and I were friends.

When I was out of school and married, I had many animals: cats, horses, gerbils, dogs, rabbits, you name it — they were part of my family. I found that all of the animals gave me much pleasure and unconditional love. That doesn't mean they don't do things that rattle you. Have you ever yelled at a dog to have him come lay at your feet five minutes later with no animosity — just giving back pure unadulterated love?

So when my friend Cheyanne asked if I would do a foreword for her book, Australian Tea Tree Oil for Animals, I was delighted. Cheyanne has raised horses and dogs and cared for them for many years. Her devotion and holistic treatment for her four-leggeds is truly inspiring. One who cares for animals is indeed a caring person in life.

My introduction to tea tree oil came in 1986. I initially became an importer of tea tree products. In 1990, I made a decision to self-publish a book on tea tree oil and human uses. I was never successful in obtaining enough information on tea tree oil and its uses in the care of animals until I met Cheyanne.

Australian tea tree oil has so many uses, it has been coined the "medicine kit in a bottle." Tea tree has many uses for horses and farm animals as well as small animals. There's an inspiring story about a milking goat that developed gangrene. After exhausting all the medical routes, the owner thought about shooting the goat. One day a friend suggested soaking the goat's leg in a bucket of warm water with tea tree oil added. The goat's leg healed in two weeks and is still healthy to this day.

The botanical name for tea tree oil is *Melaleuca alternifolia*. Tea tree is a member of the Myrtle tree family. There are over 150 species of tea trees -- the Melaleuca alternifolia being the most valuable because of its highly effective antiseptic, antibacterial, and fungicidal properties. Although clinical data using tea tree oil is sketchy, this book will give you impressive anecdotal information that shows tea tree oil to be very effective for a number of animal ailments. Tea tree oil is four to five times stronger than other household disinfectants, stings far less and has relatively low toxicity.

To emphasize the value of tea tree oil when treating serious wounds, the following testimony credits the oil with saving a mare's life.

> "On New Year's Eve, a mare of mine had an operation on her shoulder requiring stitching. Within a week, the stitching had busted open and the wound was infected with staph. The wound was deep, through the flesh and muscle, and about the size of a bread and butter plate.
>
> The vet gave the mare very little chance of surviving and they couldn't stitch the wound and he said the staph infection would spread to her blood system. I started to spray tea tree oil directly on the wound and within fourteen days, the mare was left with only a 1-2 inch scar, completely healed. The proud flesh was not burnt by the oil and I cannot believe its healing properties. My vet and other local vets were amazed and said they want copies of my photos as well so they can begin recommending it to customers."

While living in Arizona, I came across several incidents involving horse injuries. A horse developed a sarcoid, a viral condition in which a large hump appeared as a black bump. Every time the horse was ridden the rubbing of the saddle caused irritation and bleeding. The owner applied tea tree oil directly to the virus and within a short time, the sarcoid dried up and flaked off. Traditional treatments for sarcoids would be injections with the actual virus into the horse. The virus usually comes back.

Another incident involved a bruised hoof. The leg was treated with Epsom salts and tea tree oil. Within three days the inflammation and bruising were greatly reduced and the horse was able to apply full pressure on the leg.

Apparently horses get ingrown hairs too. If a saddle pad is placed on the horse against the grain of the hair, it creates an abrasion which may cause ingrown hairs. Rubbing several drops of tea tree oil into the ingrown hairs will keep infection from occurring and allows the ingrown hairs to work their way out.

When I spoke with groomers and trainers on an Arabian horse farm, I was told that the horses are in their stalls for 22-23 hours a day, and have a tendency to develop a fungus. By applying the oil directly to the infected area, the fungus dries and flakes within a matter of days. It appears to work equally well as a fly repellent, especially around the horses eyes, face and body.

More people are finding out about the remarkable success with tea tree oil, and are treating large and small animals. I feel confident that tea tree oil will become more known and used as time goes on.

At this time tea tree oil only comes from Australia. Currently between 80-100 tons of the oil are being imported into North America. The industry is growing so rapidly that I believe tea tree will become as popular as aloe vera.

Cheyanne West has bred and trained large animals for years. This guide will give readers the opportunity to learn more about this amazing essential oil — "wonder from down under" — and its extensive uses to treat a myriad of problems. Thank you Cheyanne for your valuable contribution in the realm of natural medicine for our four-legged friends.

Cynthia Olsen
Author and Researcher
February 1998

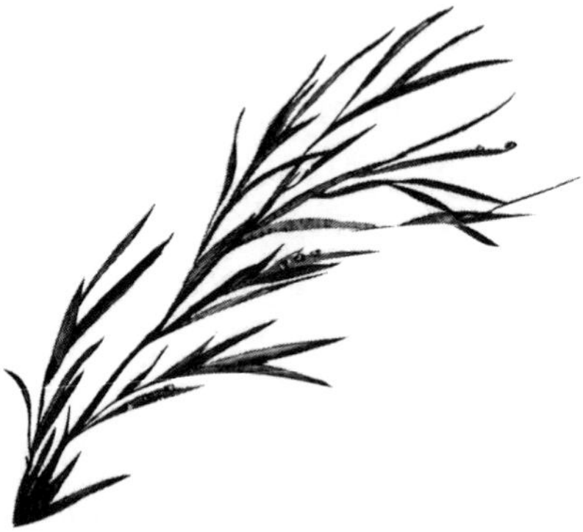

Preface

My introduction to the uses of tea tree oil came in the mid 1980's when a good friend of mine, Char Chambers, discovered this wonderful oil and later became a distributor.

One summer afternoon, Char came over excited about finding tea tree oil and explained all of the wonderful uses it had in the home. We spent the next hour or so pouring over the literature she had received and discussed the many other possible uses it may have. I purchased a small bottle of the tea tree oil concentrate and some hand cream that day. Over the next month, I used the hand cream regularly with much delight. Living in the mountains of Colorado and having numerous livestock, my hands would usually become chapped from the dry, cold winters. The tea tree oil offered much relief.

Over the course of the next 10 years, I began to use tea tree oil on my animals for such things as cuts, scrapes, to clean the insides of my animals ears, etc, and began documenting all of the uses I had discovered. I keep a log for each one of my animals — when they were de-wormed, vaccinated and what treatments I used on what ailments they had. As I reviewed these files, I was surprised to find just how many times I had used tea tree oil over the years.

I recommended it to friends for personal uses as well as to friends who had animals or whose children were in 4-H. I asked them to keep a log as well on how many times they used tea tree oil and for what situations.

Many years later, I met Cynthia Olsen, in Pagosa Springs, CO. As we got acquainted she told me of the books she had published on tea tree oil. In one of our conversations, I casually mentioned that I had had some real success using tea tree oil on animals. It was a year or two later that Cynthia approached me about writing a chapter in her book, *Australian Tea Tree Oil Guide - third edition*. Then ultimately she asked me to write this book on the uses of tea tree oil for animals. I did a lot of research in writing this book, not only drawing from my own experience and notes, but from the experiences of many other friends and acquaintances.

May I say that the treatments offered here in this book are relayed to you through experience. Not all animals react the same to tea tree oil or its treatment. The conditions outlined in here are informative and educational and by no means offer to prescribe or diagnose. Tea tree oil and other alternative therapies are not a substitute to good veterinarian care. However, tea tree oil does offer an alternative, in many situations, to using harsh chemicals or other abrasive treatments on your animals. If any condition persists, consult with your veterinarian.

I hope you have positive results with tea tree oil and that this book offers some insight into what this marvelous oil can be used for.

Cheyanne West

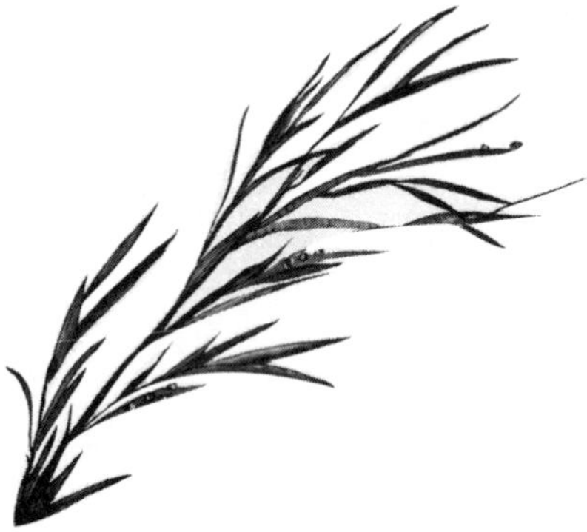

Introduction

*O*ver the past few years, tea tree oil has become more and more popular as a personal antiseptic and has gained recognition in commercial products such as shampoos, lotions and creams, acne treatments, household cleaners, deodorants, insect repellents and soaps. Each year more and more uses are being discovered for this marvelous oil and new products now offer tea tree oil as an ingredient.

Tea tree oil is a non-irritant antiseptic, fungicide and disinfectant of great repute. It is wonderful as a cream for dry, cracked skin, in a vaporizer for congestion and in shampoo for ticks, fleas and fungus. Tea tree oil is invaluable in any medicine chest in the house or in the barn as an antiseptic.

When the oil is applied to a pus-filled infection, it will clean the area, dissolving the pus without irritating the surrounding tissues. It is used topically for infections, for skin fungus, for yeast infections, poison oak or ivy, on warts and a variety of dermatitis in both humans and animals. Tea tree oil is also great as a liniment for sprains and muscle aches and, combined with other ingredients, can be used as an after-bath body brace for yourself and/or your horse.

The Australian tea tree, *Melaleuca alternifolia*, grows only in a small area of Southeast Australia. It grows along the rivers and in and around swampy grounds. The feather-like leaves secrete the oil-like droplets. The leaves are harvested and cooked in stills which extract more oil. Today, new plantations of *Melaleuca* nurseries are providing the major source for this incredible oil.

Tea tree oil products can be found at many local health food stores or through independent distributors. For those interested in learning more about Australian tea tree oil and its history, there are several excellent books available through **Kali Press** PO Box 2169, Pagosa Springs, CO 81147-2169, (970) 264-5200, (888)999-KALI (see order page at back of book).

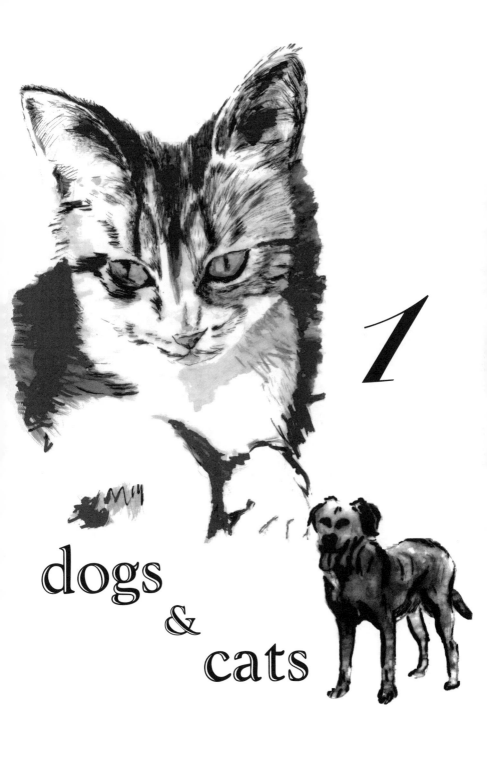

1

dogs & cats

Introduction

*F*or many of you, tea tree oil has become a household name. Over the years it has appeared in many commercial products for animals such as shampoos, lotions and creams, insect repellents and soaps.

Tea tree oil is a non-irritant antiseptic, fungicide and disinfectant of great repute. This first aid handbook offers a recipe for you to make your own salve (See Section 3) as well as many uses for tea tree oil straight or in a diluted form. I have used tea tree oil on both of my dogs and cats with wonderful results. For many years I raised Rottweilers, having as many as 9 adult dogs at one time. Though I am down to one now, who is presently 12 years old, I still use the tea tree oil to maintain the inside of his ears and for any insect bites he may acquire during our walks in the mountains. Whether you use this wonderful oil on yourself or on your dog, cat or horse, it is a valuable medicine in any home.

General Skin Conditions (Dermatitis)

Tea tree oil is very helpful in treating all kinds of skin conditions. A cat's skin is more sensitive than a dog's so it is advised that you dilute the tea tree oil in a mixture of water or oil before treating a cat. Tea tree oil or a diluted mixture can be applied to a cotton ball and dabbed straight onto wounds, bites, rashes, vaccination sites and stings. This will not only aid in healing the area but also soothe any discomfort there may be.

Strays or animals in poor condition are prime candidates for various types of dermatitis. These animals should be bathed thoroughly, removing any long hair and scrubbing the affected area with a mild soap and water. Depending on the seriousness of the condition, rub the tea tree oil into the affected area twice a day until the condition has improved. It is always best to keep the animal isolated in a pet cage or carrier to monitor the condition and prevent contagious conditions from spreading (also see minor cuts and abrasions for further instructions).

A cat's skin is very sensitive, so always dilute the tea tree oil with water or oil before treatment.

Ears

I have used tea tree oil very successfully over the years for cleaning the insides of the ears of both of my dogs and cat. Although it is not recommended that you drop tea tree oil directly into the ear canal, you can put a drop or two onto a cotton swab and squeeze off the excess and swab out the inside of the ears. Use this method daily for very dirty ears, for ear mites or waxy build up. The tea tree oil serves to clean and disinfect the inside and outside of the ears.

Sunburn

Although sunburn is rare in cats, it does occur in dogs, usually on the snout or nose area.

It is best to keep the sunburned area moist since it can be very painful. Mix equal parts of vitamin E oil and tea tree oil and apply in the evening to help soothe the burn. Keep the animal out of the sun as much as possible. If you can, keep the area covered when exposed to the sun with a zinc oxide cream or sun screen.

Warts

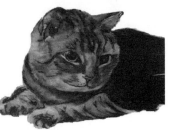

Warts are not particularly common. Older dogs and cats are most likely to develop them when they do occur. Although most warts clear up in time, they can cause discomfort if they itch or bleed.

Dab tea tree oil directly onto the warts to help

soothe the pain and dry the area. It may take a few weeks of daily application to clear up this condition.

Ringworm

Ringworm, lice and mange usually affect unhealthy animals whose immune systems are weakened. All three conditions are contagious to humans as well as to other animals.

Ringworm is more common in cats than dogs. It begins as a spot which spreads out, creating a ring-shaped sore. The hair sometimes breaks off and creates a course stubble. On cats, it may appear as gray patches of short, thin hair.

To treat ringworm, clip away the hair around the affected area and scrub with a mild soap and water. Apply tea tree oil or a mixture directly onto the area with a cotton ball or swab. Do this twice a day for at least one week. This condition can be difficult to clear up, so stay with it. The cat or dog should not be allowed to roam freely in the house but should be confined in a kennel or carrier until the condition is cleared up. Disinfect the kennel or carrier each time you treat the animal. Disinfect scissors, grooming tools and treatment area using bleach, alcohol or tea tree oil.

Farm dogs and cats are most at risk for lice and can infest other animals.

Lice

Lice infestation is more common in the winter months and in certain areas of the country. They are most active at the end of autumn. Dogs and cats who are around farm animals are the most at risk. Although lice do not live long on their host, there is a danger of infestation to other animals. As with mange and ringworm, the animal should be isolated during treatment.

Wash the cat or dog thoroughly with a mild soap and water. You may also add 1/4 teaspoon of tea tree oil to your pet's shampoo. Regular use will help maintain good hygiene. Clip off any excess hair or shave the affected area. Mix one teaspoon of tea tree oil with one cup of warm water. Put this mixture into a spray bottle and shake well before each use. Spray the affected areas on the animal and allow it saturate. Let the animal stand with the solution for up to ten minutes. Use a paper towel to pat the area dry and dispose. Use a cotton ball saturated with tea tree oil on the stubborn areas. Treatment should be repeated daily for at least one week or until signs of the lice are gone. It is best to keep the animal isolated during treatment to prevent further spreading of the lice.

Mange

There are several types of mange that can infect dogs and cats.

Sarcoptic mange is caused by a scabies mite that burrows into the skin. Demodetic mange is caused by a microscopic mite that lives in the hair follicles. These are more common in dogs and rarely seen in cats. Animals that have generalized mange are more susceptible to other serious illnesses and must be treated carefully to restore health. If this is neglected, the skin may become thickened and rigid.

If mange is neglected, your dog's skin may become thickened and rigid.

As with ringworm and lice, bathe the animal thoroughly with mild soap and warm water. Clip away any excess hair or shave the area. Combine one teaspoon of tea tree oil in a cup of water and put mixture into a spray bottle shaking with each use. Spray the animal down thoroughly and allow them to stand for up to ten minutes. Use a paper towel to dab off the excess moisture, then dispose. Saturate a cotton ball with tea tree oil and dab onto the stubborn areas. This treatment should be repeated daily for at least one week or until signs of the mange are gone. Keep the animal isolated during treatment and disinfect the kennel or pet carrier as well. This condition can be stubborn. You may need to contact your veterinarian for further suggestions.

Ticks and Fleas

To remove ticks that have attached themselves to your cat or dog, use a dropper to put one drop tea tree oil onto the tick and wait a minute or two. Then, using a pair of tweezers, grab the tick and pull gently for about 5-10 seconds, then pull it out. This action should pull the head out too. If it doesn't, the head will remain in the skin and fester. To cut down any potential swelling and infection, put another drop of tea tree oil onto the site and rub in (A note of caution: it is best to remove ticks wearing gloves, or by tweezers or by placing your hand into a plastic bag before grabbing the tick. Using a barrier between you and the tick will help prevent any exposure to tick fever, etc.

Caution:
When pulling ticks off your dogs and cats, always have a barrier between your hand and the tick itself. Lyme's disease and Rocky Mountain Tick Fever can be transmitted.

Fleas can cause a lot of problems. Dogs can chew raw spots on their skin, and cats and dogs can become infected with tape and/or roundworms from fleas. Adding nutritional yeast and garlic to the diet can help repel fleas as well as regular bathing with tea tree oil added to your pets' shampoo.

If you have seen signs of fleas on your pet, bathe your animal with mild soap and warm water and clip away hair around any rashes or existing "hot spots" (hot spots occur when a flea has chewed on an area of the skin until it is raw). Mix one teaspoon of tea tree oil into one cup of water, shake and spray the animal down well. Allow to stand for a few minutes. Then saturate a cotton ball with tea tree oil and dab onto the raw areas. It is a good idea to bathe and spray your pet outdoors, if possible, to prevent fleas from jumping off onto your carpets. With this condition, vacuum often and purchase a generic flea collar and put it into the vacuum cleaner bag to kill any ticks and fleas or their eggs that you may pick up from your carpet or furniture.

Handy Hint:

Place a generic flea collar inside your vacuum cleaner bag to kill any ticks or fleas or their eggs that may have dropped onto the carpet or furniture.

Abscess and Puncture Wounds

Abscesses in dogs and cats are usually a result of a fight. These are more common in cats. Because of a cat's needle-like claws and teeth, the wounds inflicted are quite narrow and deep, and the skin can heal rapidly over the surface, trapping bacteria and foreign matter in the wound. Most wounds can be found at the base of the tail (indicating the cat is retreating from the fight) or around the head or front legs (indicating the cat was aggressive). Abscesses in dogs are more commonly caused by plant awns, burrs, or foxtails that get trapped in the hair and work their way through the skin. These are most commonly found between the toes and around the ears or hind legs. Abscesses can also occur in other areas such as the anus and inside the mouth (when located in the mouth they are commonly referred to as mouth ulcers).

Always consider the severity of the wound: stitches may be required in some cases or other treatment considered.

Most abscesses look like an infected boil and will usually drain. Those areas that drain but do not heal well are called fistulas and are usually an indication that there is foreign matter in the abscess. Clean the area thoroughly with warm water and a mild soap. If the abscess has not burst, keep the area clean and put 1-2 drops of tea tree oil directly onto the site. Most of these wounds are sensitive to the touch. If the abscess is draining, keep the area clean. The tea tree oil will dissolve the pus without irritating the surrounding tissues.

Depending on the situation, abscesses should be cleaned and treated at least twice a day. You can put tea tree oil in a small travel-size spray bottle and spray the area if necessary; however, do not store a concentrated oil in a plastic bottle for a long period of time. Using a spray will be helpful in accessing mouth ulcers and hard-to-reach areas as well.

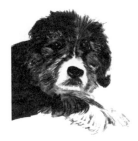

For general wounds, minor cuts and abrasions, you can apply tea tree oil directly onto the wound to aid in healing. It is best to dilute tea tree oil when applying it to a cat's wound because its skin is so much more sensitive.

I have a brave young Himalayan cat. She was given to me already declawed and spayed. On occasion, she seems to find it necessary to take on the barn cats. Unfortunately, she always comes in with tufts of hair missing around her tail and back legs, not to mention the cuts and the occasional puncture wounds she receives. I have always found it better to use a few drops of tea tree oil in water and wash the wound first or use the tea tree oil salve I have made on these minor cuts rather than to apply the tea tree oil directly to the skin. Though she may lick it off, the salve recipe does not include enough tea tree oil to hurt them internally.

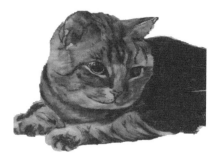

Insect Bites, Rashes, Hives and Liniments

Tea tree oil can be used on a variety of insect bites or stings. Always remember to remove the stinger, then put a drop of tea tree oil onto the site to soothe any pain and swelling. For minor scratches, hives and rashes, use a light mixture of 1 teaspoon of tea tree oil in one quart of water and saturate a rag to wash or just use it as a general rinse for the area. This method can be used for minor allergic rashes and hives, repeating until the condition has cleared.

Tea tree oil is a natural insect repellent. It can help repel fleas, ticks and some parasites as well. Many insect repellents on the market today contain tea tree oil. You can make your own by mixing one teaspoon of tea tree oil in one cup of water. Put this mixture into a spray bottle and use this to spray your dog or cat before they go outside. This mixture may also be used to spray pet carriers or bedding to help keep the area free of pests. Keep in mind that this is the strongest recipe mentioned, always avoid the eyes when spraying any pet with this mixture. Spray your hand or a rag then wipe around the eyes and over the snout and chin area.

Dental Problems

During the years of raising numerous litters of puppies, I went to the super market and became acquainted with the butcher. Every Monday afternoon he would save a bag or two of beef bones for me. He would give me full sized shank bones for the adult dogs (whom I referred to as the "kids", since I have no children of my own) and include a bag of smaller ones for the puppies (whom I affectionately called the"kidlets"). This was a big treat when I returned home. Everyone would get their bone and run off into some distant corner of the farm and spend the next several hours gnawing away at their treat. Molly, one of my adult dogs would always run and find a place to bury her bone then spend the next few hours tormenting the others into giving up their bone to her. On occasion one of them did and she would grab that and bury that one as well and repeat the process all over again. Often I would find ripened and rotted bones in my garden. I had two adult dogs in particular that would end up with very red sore gums from the hours of chewing. The tea tree oil worked really well in clearing up this condition. I would put a drop or two of tea tree oil onto a cotton swab and dab it onto the sore gum line once or twice a day. They were never particularly fond of the taste but it offered relief from the pain and helped heal the area.

Tea tree oil can also be very helpful after a dog has returned from having their teeth cleaned by the veterinarian. Many times the gums are left swollen, red and sometimes still bleeding. Again, swabbing them with a bit of tea tree oil usually clears up the condition within a few days.

For dogs who have had a tooth pulled or it has broken off, I use the same method to aid in healing the wound without infection.

With regards to cats, I have had no cooperation at all in treating any mouth sores. In fact the one time I did try it, I ended up treating the scratches on my hands and arms over the next few days instead. So I offer this advise. Tea tree oil, diluted 2-3 drops in one teaspoon of water and the swab dipped into that mixture does work on cats, however, have someone else hold the cats feet and by all means wear gloves!

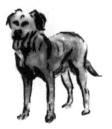

Home Uses & Disinfectants

Tea tree oil acts as a great disinfectant and fungicide. Add 1 tablespoon of tea tree oil to one quart of water and immerse grooming tools, collars, blankets, kennel pads etc. Allow them to soak overnight. For the blankets, sweaters and kennel pads, after soaking, pour out water and put items into the washing machine and wash as normal. This is especially important if you have had a sick animal and do not want anything to spread.

You can use this same mixture and put it into a spray bottle and disinfect pet carriers, wire kennels or spray directly onto the concrete or chain link kennel areas and then hose down. This will not only add a more pleasant smell to the area but will also help cut down on bacteria (see Mixtures, Recommendations & Precautions for further instructions).

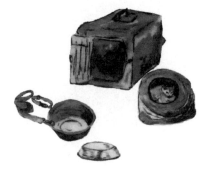

Recommended Mixtures for Dogs & Cats

STRONG MIXTURE: For disinfecting brushes, grooming tools that have been contaminated, spraying down kennels, pet carriers and for washing contaminated towels, sweaters, blankets, pads etc. use 1 tablespoon tea tree oil to 1 quart of water. Put the mixture into a bucket or a squirt bottle and spray the area. Use 2-3 tablespoons of tea tree oil directly into your washing machine load to disinfect larger quantities of towels, pads and blankets. Let them sit in the tub of water for at least 1 hour, then wash as directed.

MEDIUM MIXTURE: 1 tablespoon of tea tree oil added to 2 quarts of water . Use this mixture for general weekly or monthly cleaning of grooming tools, kennels etc.

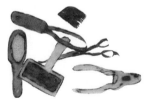

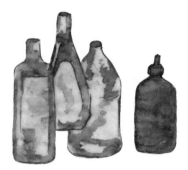

LIGHT MIXTURE: 1 teaspoon of tea tree oil added to 1 gallon of water or 5-20 drops of tea tree oil in shampoos, coat sheen, or conditioning products. Use this light mixture for rinsing and cleaning scratches or for skin conditions that are not serious. (Note: when you need to mix tea tree oil with other oil, we recommend a non-fragrant oil such as vitamin E or even a sunflower seed oil).

PRECAUTIONS
AVOID ANY CONTACT OF TEA TREE OIL WITH THE EYES. DO NOT DRINK TEA TREE OIL. KEEP OUT OF REACH OF CHILDREN.

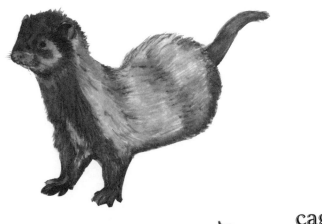

2

OTHER HOUSEHOLD ANIMALS

*T*ea tree oil can be used effectively for other domestic animals such as rabbits, birds, guinea pigs, hamsters, gerbils, ferrets and even pot bellied pigs. Although there may be some cases in which Tea tree oil can be used for reptiles, I do not have enough experience with these pets to have used tea tree oil beyond what is mentioned here.

I was pleased to discover how many other household pets could benefit from the medicinal uses of tea tree oil. Having birds, hamsters and the like in my own life of a farm, I fast became the neighborhood paramedic of sorts. One day a neighbor friend called to say that Mini-Pig, (a potbellied pig she had) got into a scrap over her dinner bowl with a 10 month old Australian Shepherd. I don't know who scared who most when Mini-Pig went to screaming but the dog panicked and bit Mini-Pig on the back and created quite a wound. After Mini finished her food, we gathered her up and cleaned off the cut with soap and water and put tea tree oil on the wound. Surprisingly, the cut healed without infection within 3 days. Needless to say, the dog and Mini-Pig are now in separate pens when they eat!

Tea Tree Oil for Caged Birds

Tea tree oil can be used in many different treatments for birds as well as an effective disinfectant for cages, toys and other items.

All birds require good nutrition as well as good hygiene to live a healthy life. Caged birds are no exception, and they are also susceptible to certain types of mites and parasites. Feather picking is a frustrating syndrome characterized by loss of or damage to the feathers from the neck down. Feather picking is usually the sign of some other underlying problem and this should be addressed by your veterinarian.

Other skin conditions can include papillomas which are warty-type proliferations that can affect some bird species. These pink to white growths are often covered with dry brown crusts that can be easily removed with surgery. They commonly appear on the neck, toes, and lower beak. It is best to use a diluted form of tea tree oil for the neck or toe area and to avoid treating the beak. For treating open wounds, it is best to use a diluted form of tea tree oil. Clean the wound with warm soapy water and rinse. Allow this to dry. Use 3-5 drops of tea tree oil in 1/4 cup of warm water. Saturate a cotton ball or cotton swab and squeeze out the excess. Dab this onto the wound. Repeat for two to three days until wound begins to heal.

Safety Suggestion: *Keep your cage free of sharp objects or loose wire and away from drapery cords and other potentially dangerous household items.*

Most wounds on birds usually do not bleed freely. If this does occur, immobilize the bird and locate the site. Apply pressure with your fingertip for about a minute or so. Use a clean cotton swab to clean away and assess the situation. The most common types of wounds found in birds are punctures and lacerations. Wounds are commonly caused by a piece of wire jutting out in the cage or an attack by another bird (or cat) or flying into an object. Punctures are generally painful and may or may not be accompanied by bleeding. Carefully pluck away the feathers from the site by holding tightly to the base of the feather with your fingers. As with any puncture on an animal, gently see that there is no foreign body embedded in the site. Clean the area well with soap and water and rinse. Dab dry with cloth or cotton swab. Put 3-5 drops of tea tree oil into a 1/4 cup of water. Saturate a cotton ball or swab, squeeze off the excess, and dab directly onto the cut. If the wound begins to bleed, apply pressure using a clean finger, with or without a gauze pad. Apply the pressure for about a minute or so. If the puncture appears to be deep, it would be best to take the bird to your veterinarian for further examination. The tea tree oil will aid in healing and soothe any pain or irritation involved. You can use the same methods for lacerations as well. This can also be applied to sore toes or bleeding toe nails. It is best not to use tea tree oil on the beak or around the eyes or face of a bird. Birds do heal fairly quickly, so repeat the treatment daily until wound is healed.

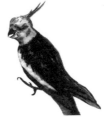

I once had a lovely bright yellow talkative parakeet named Bird. Bird was the busiest creature I ever had. She would stand screeching at the wild birds who came to the feeder near the window by her cage. When she was outside of the cage, she investigated everything and quickly became a thief. I found an assortment of items at the bottom of her cage that she had absconded with. One day she did something to tear her toenail. Knowing how painful it is for me, she stood holding up the one leg that displayed a drop of blood on one of the toes and proceeded to scold me like I wasn't doing something fast enough to fix her wound. Holding her with one hand, I cleaned the toe off as she softly closed her eyes. I put 2 drops of tea tree oil into a tablespoon of water and dipped a cotton swab in this mixture and placed that on her ailing toe. She opened her eyes and perked up then shut them again as the tea tree oil began to soothe the pain.

Disinfecting Items

Cages should be cleaned from top to bottom and perches cleaned and rotated at least once a week.

Always line the bottom of your animals' cage with a white paper towel or cloth instead of newspaper - ink can be harmful.

Food dishes and water dishes should be cleaned and disinfected as well. Toys should be either cleaned or rotated on a daily basis. This can be done with tea tree oil by adding 1/4 teaspoon to a cup of water and pouring that into a spray bottle and spraying the cage down thoroughly, let it set for a few minutes then rinse well with tap water and dry. Soak dishes in a water-filled margarine bowl (excellent small bird dishes), add a drop or two of soap and add 10 drops of tea tree oil to the water. Wash well, then rinse and let dry. Line the bottom of the cage with a white paper towel or cloth instead of newspaper, as the ink can prove harmful to your feathered friend.

Guinea Pigs

Guinea pigs are susceptible to several skin disorders that can be treated with diluted doses of tea tree oil. Pododermatitis are moist ulcerated skin lesions that occur on the feet, usually caused by trauma or from wire floors and from being kept in an unhealthy environment. Clean and sanitize the cage by using 1/4 teaspoon of oil in a cup of water and pour this into a spray bottle and spray the cage down thoroughly. Other items such as bowls and feeding dishes should also be disinfected as well. Rinse the cage and bowls thoroughly and let dry. Clean feet thoroughly with warm soapy water and rinse. Dilute 3-5 drops of tea tree oil in a 1/4 cup of water and using a cloth or cotton swab, coat the feet well with this mixture, then let set for a minute or two. Rinse feet and dab dry with paper towel and return guinea pig to a clean cage. Repeat 2-3 times per week until the problem clears up.

Hair loss can occur anywhere on the body but is usually caused by skin parasites, fighting, ringworm, or pregnancy. Chewing or "barbering" as it is sometimes called is annoying, not only to the animal, but to the keeper as well.

Ringworm includes hair loss with crusts usually located on the head, ears or back. Ringworm is caused by a virus and is contagious to other pigs as well.

Mange (caused by mites) produces intense itching, hair loss on the face and ears, and sometimes can cause seizures. This is also very contagious to other pigs. Fleas, ticks, and lice cause itching and hair loss as well, however, mange is more intense. These skin problems can be treated by washing the pig well with warm soapy water and rinse (we recommend using latex or rubber gloves during this procedure). Clip away any hair that appears to be unhealthy. Put 10-15 drops of tea tree oil into 1/4 cup of water and saturate a couple cotton balls. Dab these cotton balls onto the affected area and let it set for a few minutes. Rinse well and return pig to an isolated and clean cage. Repeat this process until the condition has cleared. As in any skin condition with your pet, if this doesn't clear up within a week or two, contact your veterinarian for additional information. Use 1/4 teaspoon of tea tree oil in 1/2 cup of water and put this mixture into a spray bottle. After cleaning the cage or carrier and bowls thoroughly, spray these items down with the tea tree oil mixture, allow them to set a minute, then rinse them thoroughly. Dry everything off and re-line the bottom of the cage. As with other pets, it is best to use a natural paper towel and avoid using newspaper as the ink from the paper may prove harmful to your pet.

Gerbils & Hamsters

Both hamsters and gerbils can be affected with skin disorders such as mange, dermatitis, and abscesses (usually from fights). Mange appears as hair loss, scaling, or itching. On hamsters, it appears along the back and face and on gerbils it is expressed at the base of the tail and rear legs. In both animals often it is a secondary condition to other diseases. Gerbils are also susceptible to dermatitis which appear as moist skin lesions, abscesses, hair loss or abrasions which can appear on the nose. They are usually secondary to poor husbandry and sanitation or self-induced trauma or parasites.

Gerbils and hamsters can be affected with skin disorders such as mange and dermatitis which tea tree oil can easily clear up.

Remove the animal from its environment and clean the cage thoroughly with warm soap and water. Put 1/4 teaspoon of tea tree oil into 1/2 cup of water then pour this mixture into a spray bottle. After washing the cage and rinsing, spray down the cage and bowls thoroughly and let set for a minute or so. Then rinse these items well and dry. Again, as with birds, it is not recommended that you use newspaper to line the cages as the ink from the newspaper can prove harmful to your pet.

When treating your hamster or gerbil for skin problems, it is always recommended that you use latex or rubber gloves and keep animals isolated until the condition is cleared up. Wash your gerbil or hamster with warm mild soapy water and rinse. Clip away any area of hair that appears matted. Gently towel dry and allow the animal to dry off a bit. Put 3-5 drops of tea tree oil in 1/4 cup of water and saturate a cotton ball or cotton swab. Dab the affected area and wait a moment or two then rinse with a clean damp cotton ball and let dry. Return the animal to a clean cage separate from other pets to insure no one else is infected. Repeat the treatment 2-3 times per week until the condition is cleared up. Hygiene and nutrition is of the utmost importance when having hamsters, gerbils or guinea pigs as pets (Please note that these treatments can apply to pet mice and rats).

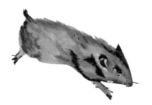

Rabbits

Rabbits can make great household pets. There are now well over 50 breeds to choose from. They come in three basic sizes, small, medium and large. Body weights can reach as much as 15 pounds. Like any small house pet, their nutrition and hygiene is of the utmost importance. Rabbits are no exception. They require a clean litter box as well as housing to help maintain good health.

Rabbits are also susceptible to fleas, skin and coat diseases, ringworm, ear-mites, mange and ticks as well as a few other problems. Tea tree oil can be used in a diluted form to treat the skin disorders as well as used as a disinfectant for their cages, bowls and litter boxes.

Rabbits are susceptible to a condition called "Sore Hocks" (a bacterial dermatitis). It appears as moist ulcerated skin lesions on the hind feet. This can be caused by trauma from wire floors, and/or environmental filth. Clean the cage thoroughly with warm soap and water and let dry. Combine 1/4 teaspoon of tea tree oil with 1/2 cup of water and pour this combination into a spray bottle. Spray cage (or carrier) down thoroughly, then rinse clean. As with other caged pets, it is best not to use newspaper to line the bottom of the cage as the ink may prove harmful to your pet. Use organic compost, paper towel or white cloth. Wash your rabbit's hind feet well with warm soapy water and rinse. Put 5-10 drops of tea tree oil into 1/8 cup of water and saturate a cotton ball. Dab onto the affected area on the feet and let it set a moment. Dab off any extra moisture and return your pet to a clean environment. Repeat this treatment 2-3 times per week until the condition is cleared up. For very serious or stubborn conditions contact your veterinarian.

Ringworm, mange, ticks and fleas can all cause intense itching, hair loss and crusty formations on various places on the body. Mange and ringworm are both contagious, as are fleas and ticks. It is best to isolate the animal during treatment. Clean and disinfect their cage and carriers using the above method. Wash the rabbit with warm soapy water and rinse and towel off. Clip away any matted hair from the area where the mange or ringworm or signs of fleas have been. Put 5-10 drops of tea tree oil into a 1/8 cup of water and saturate a cotton ball. Dab the cotton ball onto the area and let them sit a moment. Dab off excess moisture with a paper towel and dispose. NOTE: With all contagious skin conditions, wear protective gloves. It is always best to disinfect the tools you use (e.g., scissors etc.) and /or dispose of any paper towels, cotton balls etc. Do not reuse the towels until they too have been disinfected and washed. It is best to disinfect their cages each time you treat the rabbit so as not to reinfect them.

Should you encounter a tick, place one drop of tea tree oil onto the tick itself and wipe off the excess that may drip onto the hair. Wait a few moments and with a pair of tweezers or rubber gloves, grab the tick and pull steadily and gently until the tick comes out. Do not pull the tick out with your bare hands. It is best to put a barrier between your hand and the tick to prevent exposure to fevers or disease. For more stubborn ones you may have to pull harder. Then put a drop of tea tree oil onto the site to ease the pain and aid in healing.

Fleas may leave little red spots on the skin after biting. Put one drop of tea tree oil onto a cotton swab and squeeze out the excess and dab onto the sites. Fleas are not particularly fond of tea tree oil and may jump off seeking another host. If the rabbit is a house pet, I recommend purchasing a generic flea collar and putting this into your vacuum cleaner bag so when you do vacuum the house, picking up any fleas or their eggs on the carpet, the flea collar will kill the fleas captured in the bag.

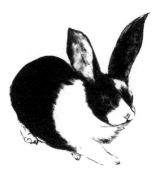

I remember one afternoon the doorbell rang and when I opened it, there was a neighborhood girl named Emily who was in tears holding her pet rabbit in her arms. "What is wrong, Emily?" I asked her. "My rabbit has bugs in his ears and my mom said that he can't come back into the house until I get them cleaned." Well, I had to hold back my smile since Emily obviously had been crying pretty hard. So Emily and I went down to the tack room in my barn and put Buddy, her rabbit, on the table where we got some water, some tea tree oil and cotton swabs and set out to clean Buddy's ears. For the next 45 minutes, Emily held tight to Buddy and told me all about what she was doing in school and how she looked forward to Buddy winning in 4-H at the county fair this year. I cleaned out the ears with soapy water then dipped a cotton swab in tea tree oil and swabbed them out real good. Though Buddy's ears were a bit red after we treated him, they were clean and Emily's mom allowed Buddy to come back into the house.

Ear mites are usually present when a rabbit shakes his head excessively, or scratches his ears. Crust or scabs have formed within the ears, making them itch. It can also be accompanied by hair loss on the head and neck. This is a very common problem in pet rabbits. Clean the ears thoroughly with warm soapy water and a cotton swab. After cleaning them the best

Never put tea tree oil full strength directly into an animal's ears, or around the eyes or mouth — it may burn the delicate skin.

that you can, the area inside the ear may appear red and raw. Put one drop of tea tree oil onto the tip of the cotton swab and squeeze off the excess. Swab the inside of the ear, being careful not to penetrate too deeply into the ear canal. Do not drop the tea tree oil directly into the ear or ear canal. Repeat every day until the condition clears up. If condition remains or becomes stubborn, contact your veterinarian for further information.

When treating any contagious skin conditions, wear protective gloves. Disinfect the tools you use (e.g., scissors etc.) and dispose of any paper towels, cotton balls etc. Disinfect and wash any towels or bedding before reuse. Clean and disinfect cages and toys each time you treat any animal so as not to reinfect them.

Rabbits are also susceptible to Pox Viruses which appears as wart-like growths on the face, legs, and feet and is sometimes accompanied by swollen eyelids, an eye discharge and subcutaneous lumps. This virus is transmitted by biting insects. Although the wart-like growths usually regress on their own, you may use one drop of tea tree oil on a cotton swab and dab this onto the area. Use a paper towel to soak up any excess. This will help minimize any discomfort the animal may have from this condition.

As with all household pets, it is always best to keep tea tree oil out of the eyes and use only diluted mixtures in the ears and around the mouth. Tea tree oil can also be used if you have clipped their nails too short causing discomfort or bleeding. Saturate a cotton ball with tea tree oil and squeeze out the excess and dab onto the affected nail, the tea tree oil will also help soothe the pain.

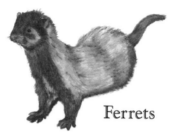

Ferrets

These mischievous little creatures are becoming more common as a household pet. Interestingly enough, they are susceptible to diseases that can effect both dogs and cats; these being the canine distemper virus and heartworm. Some ferrets have even tested positive for the feline leukemia virus. They also can contract some of the same types of intestinal parasites that affect both dogs and cats. I mention this because if you have both cats and dogs and plan to add a ferret to your family, these are things that you should keep in mind.

Ferrets are also susceptible to skin parasites, fleas, mites and ear mites. This can be detected by excessive itching, hair loss, skin or ear inflammation. They can be treated similarly as other pets mentioned in this chapter. Clean and disinfect the cage, carriers, bowls, and keep them clean at all times.

When treating your ferret for skin parasites, fleas and mites, wash the ferret with warm soapy water, rinse and towel dry. Clip away any matted hair. Put 5-10 drops of tea tree oil into a 1/8 cup of water and using a saturated cotton ball, dab onto the affected area. Allow this to dry. Return the ferret to a clean environment. If he is allowed to run loose in the house, confine him during treatment. Purchase a generic flea collar and place that into your vacuum cleaner bag and vacuum the house thoroughly. As you vacuum up the carpet or furniture, the flea collar in the bag will kill the fleas or their eggs captured in the bag.

For ear mites, clean ears thoroughly with a cotton swab. Put one drop of tea tree oil onto the tip of the swab and squeeze out any extra oil. Swab out the ear, being careful not to go to deeply into the ear canal. Do not drop tea tree oil directly into the ear canal. Should conditions persist or reoccur, it would be best to take the ferret to a qualified veterinarian accustomed to treating ferrets. You will possibly need to bring in a stool sample for further investigation concerning parasites.

Ferrets are susceptible to diseases such as canine distemper, heartworm, and in some cases feline leukemia.

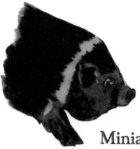

Miniature Pot-Bellied Pigs

These little guys have become the latest craze among our pet owning population. They are relatively clean and odor-free. Unlike domestic pigs, they are intelligent, easy to train and housebreak and can be very affectionate. Unlike other household pets, you will be glad to hear that miniature pot-bellied pigs are not susceptible to fleas, since they have nowhere to hide on a pigs skin! However, they are very sensitive to sunlight and cold and therefore should be kept from extremes in environmental temperatures. If allowed outside, provide shade from the intense sunlight as well as warm shelter should cooler temperatures come about.

Miniature pot-bellied pigs are susceptible to sunburn on their skin which appears as a reddening of the skin and sometimes ulcerations, depending on the degree of the burn. Provide shade for your friend if necessary, and use a light coat of the tea tree oil salve (Recipe for this is mentioned in the next section).

Seborrhea appears as dry flaky skin and can be caused by a number of conditions which include nutritional deficiencies, intestinal parasites, mange, and or unhealthy environmental conditions. The pig should be isolated from other pigs and washed thoroughly with warm soapy water, rinsed and patted dry. Mix 1/4 teaspoon of tea tree oil into 1/4 cup of water and using a saturated cotton ball, dab the reddened areas and wipe off the excess. The carrier or cage should also be disinfected.

Mange also appears as itching and small red raised bumps on the skin. Using the same method of treatment as above should help remedy the situation. However, should it become stubborn, contact your veterinarian for additional treatments.

Finally, "Greasy Pig Disease" appears as a greasy skin surface, reddened, wrinkled skin with scabs and dehydration. This condition is caused by bacteria and can be fatal in young pigs. The tea tree oil dilution will help clear up the skin condition; however, it will be necessary for you to take them to your veterinarian for additional treatment.

Cuts, abrasions, minor wounds, insect bites and stings can be easily treated with tea tree oil. Clean the area thoroughly and saturate a cotton ball with tea tree oil and squeeze out the excess. Dab onto the affected area to aid in healing and to soothe the irritation.

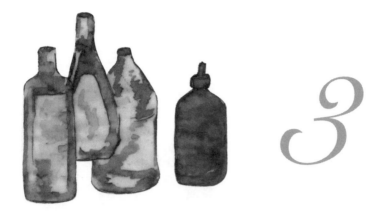

3

making your own

salves,
sprays,
washes, oils,
shampoos &
insect repellents

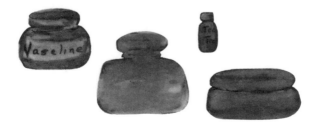

Making your own Tea Tree Oil Salve

One of the best things about tea tree oil is being able to make your own salve at home. This recipe can be doubled for larger quantities, though I have found it best to make it in the smaller quantities for easier storage.

Ingredient List:

    1 teaspoon Tea tree oil concentrate

    4 Tablespoons Vaseline or Petroleum Jelly

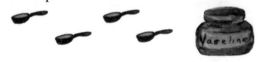

1 small jar

1 sauce pan with boiling water

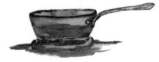

1 Put 4 tablespoons of petroleum jelly or Vaseline into a small empty jar.

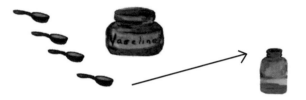

2 Take a sauce pan and fill it half way with water and bring this to a boil.

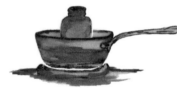

3 Put the pan onto a cool burner and place the jar of Vaseline into the pan of water, careful not to submerge the jar. The water should rise about half way up the jar. Let this stand until the Vaseline liquifies.

4 Add one teaspoon of tea tree oil to the Vaseline and stir well. Take the jar out of the pan and let it sit on the counter until the mixture starts to harden.

Place a lid on the jar and secure it tightly. This mixture can now be used on cuts, abrasions, sores and by the way, it makes a great hand cream and lip balm as well!!

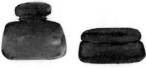

Mixtures for Horses and Other Farm Animals

Strong Mixtures: For disinfecting equipment from mites, bacteria, etc., use 1 tablespoon per quart of water. Put the mixture into a bucket or into a spray or squirt bottle and apply. Use 2-3 tablespoons in your washing machine load to disinfect blankets, etc. This mixture should be used for disinfecting only.

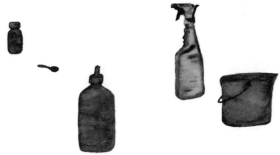

Medium Mixture: Use 1 tablespoon of tea tree oil per 2 quarts of water. This can be used for soaking cloth bandages, etc. This mixture is also recommended in the large animal section for use on

 hoofs and skin areas, unless otherwise noted.

Light Mixture: 10-20 drops or 1/4 teaspoon in 1 cup of water as noted. Use 5-10 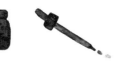 drops of tea

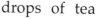

tree oil for shampoos, coat sheen or conditioning products. Use this light mixture for scratches or skin conditions that are not serious on both large and small animals.

See the end of sections 1 & 4 for additional disinfecting suggestions.

Oils

Note: if you need to mix tea tree oil with another oil, we recommend a non-fragrant oil such as Vitamin E or sunflower seed oil. Oils can be used for keeping wounds moist, or used for massage or liniments.

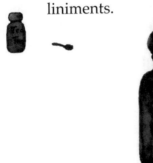

Caution:
DO NOT MIX TEA TREE OIL WITH ISOPROPYL OR OTHER RUBBING ALCOHOL.

Insect Repellent

Tea tree oil is a natural insect repellent. It repels many insects as well as flies, ticks and fleas. Many natural and herbal flea and tick products that are currently on the market now contain this marvelous oil as an ingredient. Tea tree oil dropped onto a cotton ball and applied to an insect bite or sting will aid in healing and soothing the area.

Use 1 teaspoon of the oil in one cup of
water and put this mixture into a spray
bottle. Squirt down your horse (avoiding
eyes) and don't forget to spray yourself
prior to a trail ride. Spray this same mixture onto the ear-fly-net bonnets before
you put them on the horse to aid in
warding off flies. This mixture is also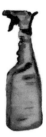
effective on summer sheets, or use it to spray the
inside of the stall or horse trailer to help eliminate
flies during travel.

Shampoos & Conditioners

There already are
shampoos on the
market containing
tea tree oil. However, if you would
like to make your own, you can
put 1/4 teaspoon of tea tree oil
into your horse's shampoo and
shake well. Tea Tree oil in the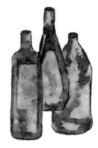
shampoo will help with many skin disorders and
aids in the overall general condition of the coat.
Apply shampoo directly, or put it into a power
spray bottle, or onto a mitt and wash the animal
thoroughly. You can also add 10 drops to your
favorite coat conditioner or coat sheen product and
spray. The tea tree oil will aid in the shine as well
as act as a general light insect repellent.

4

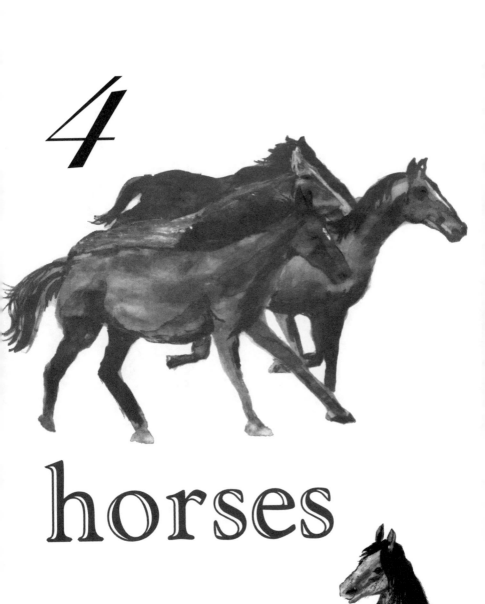

horses

Introduction

*S*ince the mid 1980's I have used tea tree oil on each of my horses. I have used it as a general antiseptic for wounds, as a liniment, and a disinfectant. I have had good luck when I used it on summer sores, and in the ears of the horses who seem particularly sensitive to flies or gnats. Whatever you choose to use this for, I have found it always beneficial to have a jar of the salve around for cuts, wounds and abrasions.

Skin Conditions

There are a number of conditions where tea tree oil can be applied to a cotton ball and dabbed straight onto a wound. It soothes the effects of insect bites, rashes, vaccination sites and stings. For sensitive open wounds, lacerations and abrasions, tea tree oil straight onto the site may cause irritation and you may encounter some resistance during treatment. You will need to use your judgment in each situation. It will be handy for you to put 1/4 teaspoon of tea tree oil in your horse shampoo (and shake) so that upon regular bathing, the tea tree oil will aid in maintaining a healthier coat. The following applications of tea tree oil are only a general guide.

Ears

In the summertime particularly, the inside as well as the outside of horses' ears can become inflamed due to gnats and flies. Before applying tea tree oil, clean the ears thoroughly to remove any dirt or crusting. Let the area dry. Put 2-3 drops of tea tree oil on a cotton ball or flannel cloth and wipe the inside of the ears well. This will act as an antiseptic, healing and soothing the irritated area. It will also act as a fly repellent. Repeat treatment every day or every other day as needed until the area is healed. A very light coat of the tea tree oil salve can be applied as long as it is a very light coat so that the heat of the sun does not cause the Vaseline mixture to drip down into the ear canal.

Do Not drop tea tree oil directly into the ear canal -it will burn the sensitive skin

Dermatitis

Horses that have not received proper care or are in poor condition resulting from poor hygiene are candidates for various types of dermatitis. These animals should be put into a dry clean area or stall. After bathing the horse thoroughly, remove any long hair and scrub the affected areas with mild soap and tepid water. Depending on the condition, tea tree oil can be applied to a cotton ball and rubbed into the affected area twice a day until the condition has cleared. It is best to keep the animal isolated to allow the condition to be supervised or monitored and to prevent any contagious conditions from spreading. Provide plenty of fresh clean water and proper feed. Consult with your veterinarian for further information on a good de-worming program as well as any other recommendations he or she may have for the care of the animal.

Ringworm

Ringworm is a contagious fungus. An affected horse should be isolated when treated, and any grooming tools that you use on this horse should be disinfected after each use. Clip away the hair around the area and scrub with a mild soap and water. Saturate 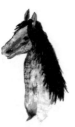 a cotton ball with tea tree oil and dab onto the affected area. This should be done 1-2 times per day for at least 7 days. This condition can be difficult to clear up, so stay with it. After the horse is clear of any signs, disinfect the stall, halter, buckets and any grooming tools that were used during treatment.

Many years ago, I had a wonderful gelding that came down with a serious case of ringworm. It covered his entire chest, midway up his neck and exhibited an occasional lesion on the back legs. This poor guy itched and lost all of the hair around the lesions. I can only gather that he contracted it at one of the many horse shows we had been to throughout the summer. I put him into the wash stall and hosed him down and washed him real good with ivory soap and betadine; then rinsed him off and allowed him to stand there until he was dry. Armed with my tea tree bottle in hand, I sprayed every lesion I could find and let him stand with the tea tree oil on him for another hour. I patted off the excess with a paper towel and put him into a clean stall away from any other horse. The lesions started out as soft swollen bumps (almost like a mosquito bite swelling) under the skin. Then the center seemed to cave in, leaving what looked like a ring under the skin. The hair began to fall out around it and the skin began to ooze. It seemed like the outbreak appeared overnight, but it took a few days to appear once I saw the bumps. I washed him for 3 straight days and repeated the tea tree oil, then washed him every other day for another week. By the end of that week, new hair began to appear and the lesions began to disappear. Though I have seen worse outbreaks that have taken much longer to clear up, this gelding of mine is now 16 years old and has never had another incident.

Lice

Lice infestation is particularly common in the winter months and in certain areas of the country. The most active signs are at the end of autumn. Lice are found generally on the neck, shoulders and under the base of the tail. Heavy infestations can include the entire body. Although lice do not survive for long on the host, there is a danger of infestation to other horses, if the brushes and blankets are shared. Wash the horse thoroughly with your tea tree oil soap and water. Put one teaspoon of the oil into one cup of water, then pour the mixture into a spray bottle. Spray the affected area until it is saturated. Let the horse stand for 10-15 minutes, then remove any excess with a paper towel and dispose. Next, saturate a cotton ball

Lice do not survive for long on their host, but there is danger of infestation to other horses.

with tea tree oil and dab onto particularly bad or stubborn areas. This treatment should be repeated daily for at least one week or until the signs of the lice are gone. Again, you may want to contact your veterinarian for further information.

Mange

Though sarcoptic mange or scabies is not as common as it once was, there is a more common mange around that is caused by a parasitic mite. There are different mites that affect different areas of the horse's body, such as the ear canal or the lower hind limbs (see leg mange). Leg mange can work up the belly and forelimbs. Though mites are barely visible to the human eye, restlessness, stamping of the feet or constant nibbling of an affected area is usually a good indication of mites. If this is neglected, the skin may become thickened and rigid.

Treatment For Mange

The horse should be isolated in a clean, dry stall away from other animals. Clip affected areas and wash thoroughly with mild soap and water. Saturate cotton balls with tea tree oil and rub into the areas. Allow this to dry. Treat the horse twice a day with the tea tree oil for 7-10 days or until signs of the mites are gone. Again, you may want to contact your veterinarian for any further instructions or recommendations. Avoid contamination by disinfecting any brushes, tools or other equipment that have been used during treatment. This includes disinfecting the stall as well.

Ticks

To remove ticks that have attached themselves to a horse, use a dropper to place several drops of tea tree oil onto each tick then wait a moment or two. Using a pair or tweezers, gently pull the tick out. This should remove the head as well. Take a cotton ball or flannel cloth that has a drop or two of tea tree oil and rub the site. This will help cut down on the swelling or potential infection. Note: Pulling a tick out with your bare hands is not recommended. There should always be a

When handling a tick, there should always be a barrier between your hand and the tick.

barrier between your hands and handling a tick. Put your hand in a plastic bag and pull the tick out, or use gloves, then dispose. I have a good friend who contracted lyme disease because she was removing some ticks from her horses with her bare hands in the field.

Warts

Although most warts clear up on their own in time, some do bleed, thereby causing some discomfort. Dab tea tree oil directly onto warts to help soothe the pain and dry up the area. This may take a few weeks of daily application. This is another situation that you could use the salve that you have made. If the warts bleed, coating them with the salve will offer some relief from the pain as well.

> *The same gelding who contracted the ringworm also got a case of the 2 year old warts. They appeared as a small cluster around one nostril then spread to cover the entire nose. They bled and it was very uncomfortable for him to eat. I coated his nose two times per day with the tea tree oil salve I made, and kept him out of the sun. The tea tree oil seemed to stop the spreading of the warts, however, it took nearly a month before they all disappeared.*

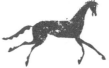

Sheath Cleaners

Most people do not care much for this job and there are many horses that don't seem to care much for it either! To make your own sheath cleaner, use about 1/4 teaspoon tea tree oil in one cup of sunflower seed oil and put it into a squirt bottle for use.

If there is only one person on hand, I suggest that you do this the first time in a stock for safety reasons. It is best to use vinyl or latex gloves when doing this job. Also, make sure your hands are warm when you start. You may not be well received with cold hands!

Put a teaspoon of this mixture into the palm of your hand and coat fingertips. This will also act as a lubricant which will be more comforting. Start with the outside of the rim of the penis and work your fingers into the sheath. Doing this gently will relax the horse, and he will start to drop. Clean out any "beans" or chunks of dirt that form and clean the area thoroughly. You may also use a bucket of warm soapy water if they are unusually dirty. Keep rinsing and repeat until clean. Don't be surprised how far up inside you can reach with your hand. Pat dry with a soft cloth. Rinse off your hands and drop some tea tree oil onto the gloves to disinfect them and coat any areas on the skin that look irritated.

Sunburn

Sunburn usually occurs on the noses of the horses who have white hair or pink skin exposed. The area should be kept moist. It is best to limit exposure to the intense sun, if possible, to aid in the healing. You can use your tea tree oil salve or mix tea tree oil with vitamin E oil and apply it in the evening to help soothe the burn. Remember this condition for the next summer. If you cannot provide cover, then cover the sensitive area with a commercial sun screen product or zinc oxide cream to protect the area from over-exposure.

I had a friend visit me one summer with her piebald paint gelding. They came from sea level to 8400 feet elevation here in the Colorado Rockies. Within the first week, my friend called me over to ask me what had happened to her horse's nose. It had begun to crack and turn a bit brown. It was indeed unsightly. I smiled and told her it was sunburn and that we needed to get something on it and get him out of the sun. Poor guy, he would hardly let us touch his nose and the cracks became so deep that they bled. It took about a week of daily treatment before it finally healed. We rode from then on only on cloudy days. This was her first experience with sunburn on her horse and next year she promises to bring sunscreen.

Wounds

For all serious open wounds, abrasions, contusions, lacerations and the like, try to determine the severity and sensitivity of the situation before applying tea tree oil straight.

Always clean the area thoroughly and apply a few drops of the oil: either straight or diluted onto a cotton ball and dab the affected area. Left to dry the tea tree oil will act as an antiseptic and aid in drying the area. For a wound that must be kept moist, mix a few drops of tea tree oil with aloe vera gel or Vitamin E oil and apply. You may also melt down 4 tablespoons of petroleum jelly (Vaseline) and add 1 teaspoon of tea tree oil to create your own salve. NOTE: Further instructions for preparing this salve as well as mixture recommendations are outlined in Section 3.

For any serious injury, always contact your veterinarian to determine if other medical attentions may be required.

Abscesses & Skin Ulcers

Abscesses and skin ulcers, whether in the mouth or on some part of the body, are painful and sensitive. A few drops of tea tree oil from a dropper put directly onto the area will help clean and dissolve pus without irritating the surrounding tissues.

Depending on the situation, these sores should be cleaned and treated at least twice a day. You can put the oil into a small travel-sized spray bottle and spray the area if necessary; however, do not store strong tea tree oil concentrate in a plastic bottle as it may deteriorate over time. Using a spray will be helpful in accessing mouth ulcers that arise from VS (vesticular stomatitis) or the herpes virus.

Dropping tea tree oil onto the abscess will help clean and dissolve pus without irritating the surrounding tissues.

Saddle Sores, Galls and Pressure Sores

These types of sores are usually caused by ill-fitting equipment or just plain abuse to an animal. Put 15-20 drops of tea tree oil into a 1/4 cup of water and saturate a piece of of cotton gauze or flannel and dab the affected area. This can be very painful for a horse. You may find it necessary to use less tea tree oil and treat the area more often. If necessary, use the salve you have made and coat the area well to help protect it. Allow the sore to heal and correct the cause of the problem. Continued aggravation of the area will only cause scarring.

Summer Sores

Summer sores are created by flies biting on one particular spot on a horse, usually on the underside of the stomach or chest area. Left untreated, they get bigger, itch terribly and develop a scab, and if severe, can eventually scar the area. Keeping a horse sprayed down with a fly repellent is one alternative. Sometimes these situations can get away from you. This happened to me with a mare I have.

We had been gone for better than a week last summer and I came home to find Katie standing off by herself and it appeared that the underside of her stomach was swollen. At first I thought she may have been kicked, but upon further inspection I quickly realized she had developed a large summer sore about the size of a tea cup saucer under there. I brought her in off of the pasture and cleaned the area with soap and water. Much of the area was raw. I dabbed hydrogen peroxide on the wound then rinsed and allowed it to dry. I put the tea tree oil salve I had made just on the wound area itself and returned her to the pasture. The next day I checked on her again and the flies had started biting the area around the wound creating another ring. I rewashed her and put almost the entire jar of salve I had made on the wound and continued about 3" past making a thick coating. It took about four days of treatment but the area healed up nicely and did not leave a scar. Sometimes these areas can become infected or so deep that the hair grows back white. Fortunately this was not the case with Katie.

General Liniment

Tea tree oil rubbed into a sore or aching muscle or sprain is wonderfully soothing and aids in attracting needed circulation to the area. Put on latex-type gloves then put a few drops of oil in your hand and/or mix the oil together with a couple drops of Vitamin E or sunflower seed (a light oil).

Insect Bites, Stings, Hives & Rashes

Anyone who has been bitten by horse flies, bees or mosquitoes, knows how irritated the skin can become. It is the same with our horses. Always clean the area and put 2-3 drops of tea tree oil onto a cotton ball and rub onto the area thoroughly. The oil will help soothe the pain and reduce the swelling caused by the sting. It will also act as an antiseptic and help clear up most of the other skin conditions that can result from the insects or irritations.

Hoof Conditions

A variety of hoof conditions can be effectively treated with tea tree oil. Put it into a spray bottle and spray areas of the hoof for conditions like thrush, quittor, greasy heel and abscesses. I use this on a preventative basis once a week and particularly after one of my horses has been trimmed or re-shod. I also recommend this same preventive treatment for horses who are prone to thrush. I know several people whose horses' feet have been saved by the repetitive use of tea tree oil when no other product worked on thrush. I think you will find it very effective.

Leg Mange

Leg mange is a condition where mites live on the surface of the skin, inhabiting primarily the fetlock region as well as the butt of the tail. The affected area can become red and ooze a serum which forms into a crust. This can be very contagious, and it is best to isolate the horse as well as disinfect the space used to clean the horse. The stall and any grooming tools such as halters, sheets, brushes, etc., should be disinfected and kept separated until the condition is cleared up (also see Skin Conditions -pg.61 for further information).

Clean the area thoroughly with mild soap and water. Protect yourself by using latex or rubber gloves. Saturate a cotton ball with tea tree oil and dab onto the affected area.

Repeat this twice a day until condition clears. You can also use a flannel cloth or cotton leg wrap soaked with tea tree oil to wrap the leg. The bandage will have to be changed 1-2 times per day. Another way to treat this is to put 1 tablespoon of tea tree oil into 1/2 cup of water and pour this mixture into a spray bottle. You may then spray the affected area as well as surrounding areas twice a day to prevent the mange from spreading. Keep this horse isolated during treatment and disinfect any tools used.

An added precaution is to burn or carry away any straw or shavings removed from the stall so that other animals do not come in contact with it. This is important for the protection of the other barn animals such as cats and dogs.

Thrush

Thrush is a foul-smelling black tarry-like discharge that can be seen in the grooves of either side of the frog area. Tea tree oil works very well on this condition. After cleaning the hoof well, you can drop the oil directly onto the affected area. Put an old cotton sock over the foot and secure. Repeat daily for up to a week or until the condition disappears. As a preventative, you can spray the foot area with a solution of 1/4 teaspoon of tea tree oil in 1/4 cup of water daily or once a week, depending on the condition. Spray the hoof with this mixture after the horse has been trimmed or re-shod to maintain a healthier hoof.

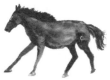

Abscesses & Punctures

Abscesses and puncture wounds can be caused by a variety of situations. At times, these can be difficult to treat and more often than not, are painful for the horse. Clean the area by scrubbing, if necessary.

For abscesses with pus, use a dropper to place a few drops of tea tree oil directly onto the area. The oil will dissolve the pus without irritating the hoof. You may cover the foot with an old cotton sock and secure with a sticky bandage to help keep the foot clean. As the wound heals, put 1 teaspoon of tea tree oil in a cup of water then put that mixture into a spray bottle, spraying the area twice a day after cleaning.

Another treatment I have used includes 1 tablespoon of tea tree oil in 1 pint of warm water to soak the foot. Tea tree oil can be dropped onto a cotton bandage, then place the bandage directly over the affected area. Wrap the foot with a bandage, then one layer of plastic wrap and secure snugly with vet wrap. Then place an old cotton sock over the foot and secure that with a sticky bandage.

I like to keep the area open. I find spraying the area with the tea tree oil mixture after cleaning and putting a sock over the foot, keeps it free of dirt. You will have to be the judge as to the severity of the condition and which treatment would work best for you. Severe punctures should be viewed by a veterinarian.

Over Reaching & Cross-Firing Wounds

Again these types of wounds can be very painful and are caused by continually striking one foot upon the other during gait. After cleaning the area thoroughly, it is best to use tea tree oil straight or in combination with water in a spray bottle. These wounds tend to be very sensitive. You may want to spray the wound first and allow the tea tree oil to soak in to take the initial pain out of the wound, before you begin to handle them. Clean the area thoroughly. Depending on the severity, you can use a tea tree oil salve or mixture on the wound, then put an old cotton sock over the foot and secure. Repeat the treatment daily until the foot is healed. The cotton sock will allow the area to breathe, and the scent of the tea tree oil will act as an effective insect repellent as well.

Quittor

Quittor is caused by an injury near or on the coronary band of the foot, which causes damage to the cartilage and the soft tissues of the heel area. It is a chronic, purulent inflammation of the lateral cartilage of the hoof wall. This area should be cleaned thoroughly, then allowed to dry. You can apply the tea tree oil salve that you have made or put 1/4 teaspoon of the oil into 1/4 cup of water then pour this into a spray bottle and spray the area. This is also a sensitive situation. It is not recommended to treat the area with the tea tree oil straight as it may cause some discomfort. Serious or neglected conditions should be viewed by a veterinarian.

Greasy Heel

Greasy heel is a form of dermatitis or inflammation of the skin, primarily in the region between the heels and back of the pasterns. It is usually found more frequently in the hind limbs rather than the forelimbs.

> My dear Katie, the mare I mentioned before with the summer sore, also acquired this condition one summer. This can be a very sensitive and very painful condition, so please use caution at the onset of treatment. She would not let me near her hind legs. So I put a 1 teaspoon of tea tree oil in a 1/2 cup of water and sprayed the back legs and allowed the tea tree oil to soothe the pain before I began to work with her.

The affected area should be cleaned and scrubbed thoroughly, then allowed to dry. Make a mixture of 1/4 teaspoon of tea tree oil in 1/2 cup of water and spray the area twice a day. The dermatitis may remain dry and cracked; if so, it is best to spray the area or apply the tea tree oil salve you have made to keep it moist. If the area oozes, it is best to keep it as dry as possible by treating it with just the oil: let it dry, then dust the area with pure corn starch. Again, this skin condition is very sensitive, and you may encounter resistance when treating it. You may need to hose off the leg(s) or soak it in a bucket (if that is possible). Whether the area is dry or moist, consider covering the foot with an old cotton sock and taping the sock to the leg. Treat the area twice a day, reapplying a new sock each time. The tea tree oil will aid in healing the area and the scent will act as an insect repellent as well.

Greasy heel is more frequently found on the hind limbs.

Farm Uses

Tea tree oil acts as a great disinfectant and fungicide. Add 1 tablespoon to 1 pint of water in a squirt or spray bottle, then shake well. Wash buckets thoroughly with soap and water, then rinse, squirt or spray the inside and bottom of the buckets and let them stand for a few minutes. Wipe out the excess with a sponge and rinse. This same mixture can be used to spray down the walls of stalls, inside water tanks, feeders or large tubs. Scrub them well and rinse.

Disinfecting Grooming Tools & Tack

Put 2 tablespoons of tea tree oil into 2 quarts of water, stir, then immerse brushes, mane and tail combs, hoof picks, curry combs, etc and allow these to soak overnight. Rinse and allow them to dry thoroughly the next day. Use this same mixture to spray down rakes, shovels and pitchforks and let them stand for 15 minutes before rinsing.

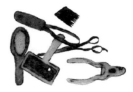

Clean and disinfect bits periodically by spraying them with tea tree oil or soaking them for a couple of hours or overnight in 1 tablespoon of tea tree oil and 1 pint of water. Rinse the bits well before using.

Today there are laundry detergents and other disinfectants and household cleaners that include tea tree oil as an ingredient. If these are not available to you, you may put 2 tablespoons of tea tree oil into the laundry tub of water with a mild soap and soak halters, saddle pads, girths and girth covers,

tail bags, shipping or skid boots and even horse blankets and sheets. Tea tree oil acts as a powerful antiseptic, proven to be 10 times stronger than the #1 chemical antiseptic, carbolic acid. If you are limited in the amount of tea tree oil you have on hand, you may put 1 tablespoon of the oil into 1 quart of water, spray the items down thoroughly and let them sit for a while before continuing to wash that load.

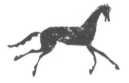

PRECAUTIONS

AVOID any contact of tea tree oil with the eyes.

Do not use or store tea tree oil around homeopathic remedies, as it will contaminate your remedy. Keep cap on tight and store in a cool, dry place.

DO NOT DRINK TEA TREE OIL - KEEP OUT OF REACH OF CHILDREN.

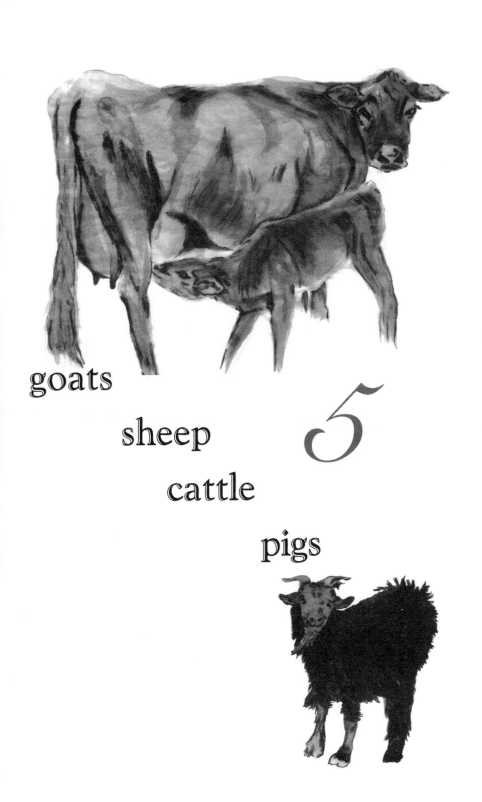

goats

sheep

5

cattle

pigs

Farm Animals

Tea tree oil has been used successfully with most farm animals. Cattle, sheep, goats and pigs have all had some benefit from its application. This chapter will outline some of the many uses it has had for these animals. It should be noted that many animals suffer from a variety of ailments and diseases. There are many times when a disease will manifest itself as a skin condition. Using tea tree oil topically will NOT cure the underlying cause of the skin condition, but rather offers support in clearing up and healing the skin condition caused by the disease. Many specific diseases should be treated by a veterinarian.

Tea tree oil can be a wonderful disinfectant. See the end of this section and section 2 for mixtures, strengths and uses in disinfecting tools, buckets, and farm equipment.

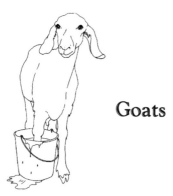

Goats

Goats suffer from a variety of ailments and diseases and there are many times when a disease will manifest a skin condition. Using tea tree oil topically will not cure the underlying cause of the skin condition, but aids in healing the lesions that appear.

"I've had milk goats for many years and I love them. They are hardy animals but things can go wrong. My favorite goat somehow got a bone infection in one leg. The vet said it's very hard to cure. We tried all the shots and pills he gave us to no avail. I tried another vet and used all the medication he gave us. No luck. Gangrene set in and we were talking about shooting her. Then a friend told me about Melaleuca — tea tree oil. I was ready to try anything! I put a few drops in a bucket of warm water and soaked her leg in it twice a day. After one week I saw improvement. After two weeks her leg was normal and hair was growing back. People couldn't believe the way she healed up. The next winter she started limping on the leg again and the hair started coming off. I soaked it in tea tree oil for a few days and she was fine."
Countryside Farm Journal, Vol..77, No. 5, September/October, 1993

Skin Conditions

There are various skin conditions to which goats are susceptible, much like sheep and cattle. They vary in severity and many respond well to tea tree oil. There are non-specific conditions which include various eczemas and photosensitization or sunburns. Specific skin conditions can include different forms of mange, ringworm, goat pox and warts. It may be beneficial to put 1/4 teaspoon of tea tree oil into your animals' shampoo. Regular bathing with this will help maintain a good coat condition. It is always recommended that you wear latex or rubber gloves when treating any skin conditions. Goats can also get a condition called Gingivitis much like humans. Put 1 drop of tea tree oil onto a cotton swab and dab the gum area. The tea tree oil will help soothe the pain and clear up the condition usually within a few days.

Eczema

Eczema is a broad term used to identify any disturbance affecting the skin. It can appear as scurfy, broken or ulcerated skin with raw or weeping areas, or what appears to be an acne-like eruption. The area should be thoroughly washed with mild soap and water and patted dry. Clip away any excess hair. Tea tree oil can be applied directly onto the area using a saturated cotton ball or cotton swab. This condition should be treated every day until it is cleared up. If it becomes stubborn or the condition worsens, consult with your veterinarian for further suggestions.

Sunburn and Photosensitization

Sunburn is more likely to be seen on goat breeds such as the Saanen and Norwegian Dairy as well as others. Photosensitization occurs world-wide and may affect many species, but is most common in sheep and cattle. It appears to be associated with the ingestion of certain plants, particularly St. John's Wort which seems to be a triggering factor. The eruptions can appear around the eyes, muzzle, teats and along the back and shoulder areas. There can be other internal derangements as well, so the severity of the condition must be considered. Provide the goat with plenty of shade while being treated. Clip away any unwanted or matted hair and clean the area. Use the tea tree oil salve that you have made and coat the area. You can apply tea tree oil directly onto eruptions that may occur. It is best to keep the oil away from the eyes. Should this condition reoccur, you should consider providing shade for the goat during the intense sunlight hours.

Abscesses

Abscesses can be acute, chronic, non-specific or specific. Specific abscesses usually arise because of secondary infection from a pus-yielding organism such as staphylococci or streptococci. Acute abscesses appear as a painful swelling and the goat is usually very sensitive to the touch. If the abscess has not erupted, you can dab tea tree oil straight onto the site using a cotton ball or swab. If it is draining, clean the area thoroughly, use a dropper to put 1-2 drops of tea tree oil onto the sight. Tea tree oil will aid in dissolving the pus

Specific abscesses usually arise because of a secondary infection from a pus-yielding organism such as staphylococci or streptococci.

without damaging the surrounding tissue. Clean the area 1-2 times a day depending on the drainage, repeat the treatment until the abscess is clear. If you encounter an abscess that you suspect is from a puncture wound, clean the area gently and check to see that the abscess itself is free of any foreign matter. Most abscesses, whether from a puncture or otherwise, are very sensitive to the touch. Tea tree oil will aid in soothing any pain or discomfort as well as assist in the healing process.

Mange

Mange is a condition that is referred to as scabies or "the itch" and is due to a mite which infests the skin causing varying degrees of infestation. There are 4 different types of mange that can affect goats. They are psoroptic mange, sarcoptic mange, demodectic mange and chorioptic mange.

Psoroptic mange in goats is much less severe than a corresponding condition found in sheep (called Sheep Scab) and is caused by a different species of mite. The goat begins to express this condition by shaking its head and/or scratching its ears. The condition may spread to the top of the head and down the neck to the shoulder area. The skin becomes dry and scurfy accompanied by itching. Left untreated, it may become infected.

Four different types of mange can effect goats: psoroptic mange, sarcoptic mange, demodectic mange and chorioptic mange.

Sarcoptic mange is a more severe type causing an extensive skin condition that is also dry and scurfy. Scabbing and itching can be more intense. If left untreated the skin can become leathery and wrinkled. Young kids are also susceptible to this condition.

Demodectic mange involves the hair follicles where mites produce what look like small abscesses. This condition can spread from the neck to the front of the legs and shoulder and on occasion can appear on the head and around the eyes. It mainly affects younger animals but is not contagious.

Chorioptic mange is sometimes known as "leg mange". Mites attack the skin of the legs causing bare patches which the goat will itch creating general irritation. The goat may be seen stamping their feet or biting at the infected area. In all cases, it is best to isolate the goat while treating them. Clean the affected area thoroughly with soap and water then rinse and clip away any matted or unwanted hair. Saturate a cotton ball with tea tree oil and dab onto the affected area as well as the out lying area. Allow this to dry. Treat the animal 1-2 times per day until the condition clears. If you are working in and around the ears, clean the ears thoroughly and put one drop of tea tree oil onto a cotton ball or cotton swab and squeeze out the excess. Then clean out the ear. Do not drop the tea tree oil directly into the ear canal. If the condition becomes stubborn or begins to get worse, contact your veterinarian for further suggestions.

Ringworm

Ringworm is a superficial fungal condition that can affect all age groups, though it is not as common in sheep and goats as it is in other species. If you do encounter this condition, you will find lesions on the head, neck and shoulder areas. It is contagious, so it is best to isolate the animal during treatment. This condition appears on the skin as a red circular ring. The skin becomes dry and scaly, but may not itch. Clean the affected area with mild soap and water and pat dry. Clip away any unwanted hair and using a cotton ball saturated with tea tree oil, dab this onto the affected area, as well as the outlying area. This should be repeated at least once a day. It can also be difficult to clear up, so stay with it.

Goat Pox

Goat pox is a vesicular and pustular condition and appears as eruptions on the skin of the udder and

Goat Pox can become serious and is sometimes fatal. Use latex or rubber gloves during treatment and contact your veterinarian for any further suggestions.

teats. Unlike other farm animals, this condition in goats can become serious. It is usually seen in the U.K. and is invariably mild in character; however, it can, in rare occasions, become fatal, so it should be watched. A specific virus is responsible for this condition and it can be contagious to other goats.

There are 4 distinct stages. The first stage known as papular is usually a small nodule which develops into the vesicular (second stage). Fluid develops within the lesion, then erupts (the third stage known as the pustular stage). Eventually, this leads to the fourth stage where a scab appears and healing has begun. The period of time from the appearance of a papule to the healing scab stage is about 8 days. There may be signs of a mild fever and the goats' teats may also become sensitive to touch; eruptions may appear. It is much like treating an abscess. First clean the area thoroughly. Saturate a cotton ball with tea tree oil and dab this onto the area if it hasn't erupted. Use a dropper to place tea tree oil onto the area after it has begun to drain. Keep the goat isolated from exposure to other animals. Use latex or rubber gloves during treatment and contact your veterinarian for any further suggestions.

Warts

Warts on the teats are caused by a virus. They are usually not serious; however, they are unsightly and prone to bleed. For those that cause discomfort, tea tree oil can be applied to the warts to help soothe the pain and sensitivity. It may take several weeks before the condition clears up. Apply the oil daily, or every other day.

Hoof Conditions

Tea tree oil can also be used on foot rot, a condition caused by contaminated soil in damp or marshy areas. This is common among sheep under these conditions and can also affect goats in varying degrees. In the early stage you may notice a slight lameness, depending on the condition. You may also notice the goat grazing frequently on its knees thereby protecting the affected foot. The horn of the hoof becomes soft and crumbly and gives off an unpleasant odor. Remove the animal from the damp environment and wash the hoof well with

Foot rot is caused by contaminated soil in damp or marshy areas.

mild soap and water. Put 1/2 teaspoon of tea tree oil in 1/2 cup of water and pour this mixture into a spray bottle. Spray the hoof well with this mixture, on the top and underneath the hoof. Keep the goat in a clean environment and treat daily or every other day depending on the severity of the condition.

Seedy Toe

Seedy toe is a bacterial condition causing pus and or oozing around the coronary band just above the hoof line. This condition is also seen in horses. The goat may become lame. Clean the area thoroughly with mild soap and water and rinse, then pat dry. Using a dropper, place the tea tree oil directly onto the site. The tea tree oil will help to dissolve the pus without irritating the surrounding tissues. You may then help to protect the area from dirt by putting an old cotton sock over the foot and attaching it with vet wrap or other type adhesive bandage around the leg. Repeat treatment 1-2 times per day depending on the severity.

Tea tree oil can also be used successfully on most cuts, wounds, bites and stings. As with any treatment procedure, clean the area thoroughly with mild soap and water, rinse and pat dry. In most cases, you can apply tea tree oil to a cotton ball or swab and dab directly onto the wound. The oil will aid in healing as well as soothe any accompanying irritation or pain. Avoid contact with the eyes.

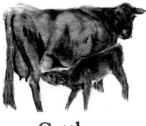

Cattle

There are many skin conditions that affect cattle for which tea tree oil can be of great benefit. As with treating any animal with a skin condition, it is always recommended that you wear latex or rubber gloves during treatment.

Sunburn and Photosensitization

Some cattle can get sunburn and photosensitization. Tea tree oil can be a very soothing treatment. Mix 1/4 teaspoon of tea tree oil to 1/3 cup of water and pour this mixture into a spray bottle. Spray the affected area (usually unpigmented areas) and avoid spraying directly into the eyes. This mixture can be used on the udder to help soothe the teats as well as during nursing. Provide shade, if necessary, for severe cases and avoid excessive direct exposure to the sunlight (if possible) until the condition clears up.

Photosensitization occurs worldwide and can affect many species. It is most common in cattle and sheep and seems to be triggered by the ingestion of certain plants such as St. John's Wort. Treat as mentioned above.

Ringworm

Ringworm is a superficial fungus that appears as a red outlined circle on the skin. There is considerable itching, and the skin becomes scaly and scurfy. Left untreated it can become crusty, hard and scab-like. The most common areas that are affected are the neck and head. Since ringworm is contagious, it is best to isolate the animal if possible. Scrub the affected area thoroughly with soapy water and rinse. Saturate a cotton ball with tea tree oil and dab directly onto the affected area. Allow this to dry. Repeat several times per week until the condition clears This condition can be stubborn, so stay with it. It is also recommended to disinfect any buckets, towels, or brushes that you may use during treatment so this condition does not spread.

Mange

Mange is sometimes called scabies or "the itch". There are three types that can affect cattle. They are psoroptic, sarcoptic and chorioptic mange. The condition is contagious and caution should be used when treating animals. They should be isolated and any grooming tools, buckets, towels, etc. should be disinfected after each use. Bedding should be changed daily and disposed of in such a manner that it does not come in contact with any other farm or domestic animals. In all three cases, latex gloves are recommended during treatment to minimize exposure.

Psoroptic mange is highly contagious and confined to cattle. It can spread by direct contact or through contaminated bedding, etc. The lesions usually begin on the shoulders and/or dorsal area of the neck and can produce intense itching. The lesions then begin to ooze serum.

There are three types of mange, sometimes called scabies or the itch, which can affect cattle.

Sarcoptic mange occurs when the mites burrow under the skin producing tunnels. The area begins to swell and becomes inflamed during the burrowing process. Itching can be severe as well. The animal begins to rub the area, leaving bare patches. Neglected cases produce thickening of the skin which becomes wrinkled into folds.

Chorioptic mange is sometimes called symbiotic or tail mange. This too is confined to cattle and is usually mild. The lesions remain small and are confined to the tail and legs. Although itching is present, it usually is not severe.

Isolate the animal and wear latex or rubber gloves during treatment. Scrub the affected area thoroughly with soap and water, then rinse. Clip away any unwanted or matted hair. Saturate a cotton ball with tea tree oil and dab the affected area as well as the surrounding area. Repeat this process, depending on the severity of the condition, at least once a day until the condition clears. Again, you will benefit by putting 1/4 teaspoon of tea tree oil into the animals' shampoo. Regular bathing with this mixture will help maintain good hygiene. It is also best to disinfect any tools used during the treatment after each use.

Cow Pox

The Cow Pox virus appears as skin eruptions that are usually confined to the teats and skin of the udder. The incubation period is from 4-7 days and much like the goat pox goes through some recognizable stages. The first stage is papular where it appears as a small nodule and lasts about two days. The second or vesicular stage appears about the third or fourth day in which the nodule fills with fluid and erupts. The vesicles contain a straw-colored fluid. This becomes pustular around the 7th or 8th day and is followed by a scab and the healing stage. Tea tree oil can be applied to these lesions at any stage which will help with the healing process and soothe pain and sensitivity. This is contagious, so it is best to isolate the animal during treatment. Using latex or rubber gloves, clean the affected area thoroughly with soap and water, then rinse. You may use 1/4 teaspoon of tea tree oil in 1/2 cup of water and pour this into a spray bottle and spray the area well. Or you may saturate a cotton ball with tea tree oil and dab directly onto the lesions as needed.

Wounds

Wounds, abscesses, lacerations, bites and stings can also be treated with tea tree oil. Wash the affected area with soap and water and rinse. Saturate a cotton ball with the oil and dab this directly onto the wound. The tea tree oil will aid in healing and soothe any pain that may occur. It will also dissolve any pus that might be present without irritating the surrounding tissue.

Abscesses

Abscesses of the foot are not uncommon among animals that are kept in unsanitary conditions. Abscesses can also occur when an animal steps on something that penetrates the sole of the foot. In either case, lameness usually appears due to severe pain. The animal will usually raise the hoof off the ground while resting. Scrub the hoof well and using a dropper put several drops of tea tree oil onto the area. The tea tree oil will help to dissolve any pus that may be present and aid in the healing process. It is best to confine the animal to a clean area during treatment.

Hoof Conditions

Foot Rot is an infection of the foot which can lead to further problems if left unattended. Lameness is present as well as an unpleasant odor. Scrub the hoof well and rinse. You can soak the entire foot in a bucket. Fill it approximately 1/3 with warm water and add 1 tablespoon of tea tree oil. Allow the foot to soak for about 5 minutes, then towel dry. Alternately, put 1 teaspoon of the oil into 1/2 cup of water and pour into a spray bottle. After cleaning the area, spray the foot down thoroughly. Keep the animal confined to a clean dry area and repeat the treatment 1-2 times per day until the condition beings to clear. Consult with your veterinarian for further suggestions.

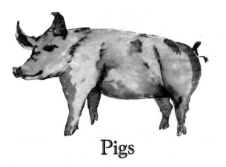

Pigs

Like their fellow miniature pot-bellied pigs, larger pigs can also benefit from tea tree oil for skin conditions. As with treating any skin condition on an animal, we always recommend that you wear latex or rubber gloves during treatment.

Skin Conditions

Abscesses are occasionally encountered and are associated with various strains of bacteria. They start out as swellings beneath the skin with the surface of the skin appearing red and discolored. The areas around the ears, shoulders and flanks seem to be the most common sites. Older animals, particularly sows, tend to develop these abscesses along the flank and on the back of the neck. At the early or acute stages of these abscesses, the site is particularly sensitive to the touch. Saturate a cotton ball with tea tree oil and dab onto the site several times per day. If caught early enough the tea tree oil may help the body reabsorb the infected site. Continue treatment, keeping the area clean while it comes to a head and drains. The tea tree oil will help soothe the pain and aid in dissolving the pus without irritating the surrounding tissue.

Candida

Candida Albicans is a fungal skin disease and appears as a circular lesion on the abdominal area and the hind limbs. The lesion may secrete a gray-ish moist fluid. Left untreated, the skin becomes thickened, hairless and ultimately becoming bluish in color. Clean the site thoroughly with soap and water and rinse. Pat dry with a paper towel and dispose. Saturate a cotton ball with tea tree oil and dab onto site several times per day until condition has cleared.

Ringworm

Ringworm is also a fungus that appears as a red circular lesion, usually causing itching. It can appear on various parts of the body, but particularly on the abdominal area. This condition is contagious, so it would be best to isolate the pig during treatment. Wash the area with soap and water and rinse. Pat dry with a paper towel, then dispose. Saturate a cotton ball with tea tree oil and dab onto the site several times per day. This condition can be stubborn, so stay with it. It is always best to wear gloves and disinfect or dispose of any towels, or brushes used during the treatment so the condition does not spread.

Sunburn and Photosensitization

Pigs that are exposed to intense sunlight may be affected with either or both of these conditions. Sunburn is most likely found behind the ears and can even effect the gait of the animal. Photosensitization occurs world-wide and is most commonly seen in sheep and cattle. The condition seems to occur at the onset of ingesting certain plants or grasses, e.g. St. John's Wort, rape and alfalfa. It seems to affect white breeds more so than breeds with pigmented areas who seem to remain unaffected This condition can appear reddish in color and go as far as peeling, thus leaving a raw area that tends to itch. Provide shade during treatment. Bathe the pig with soap and water and rinse. Use a light coat of the tea tree oil salve and repeat daily until the condition clears. If possible, provide a shaded area during intense sunny days for pigs susceptible to this condition.

Pityriasis Rosa

Pityriasis Rosa or Pustular Psoriaform Dermatitis is a condition of unknown origin. It can effect young pigs and particularly those of the Landrace breed. The condition appears as reddish papules which are hot to the touch and usually found in the abdomen and inguinal (or groin) region and sometimes on the back, though they are less severe on the back. The lesions tend to spread and change shape. There is a theory that this condition may be hereditary. Wash the affected area with soap and water and rinse. Pat dry, then saturate a cotton ball with tea tree oil, squeezing out the excess and dab this onto the affected site 1-2 times per day until the condition clears.

Foot Rot

Foot Rot is a condition that affects pigs up to six months of age, especially if they are reared inside on concrete instead of wood floors. Cracks can develop on the wall of the hoof and sometimes can involve the coronary band. A secondary infection can lead to the development of ulcers which can ultimately go deeper and involve other tissues and the bone. If neglected, this condition can lead to septicaemia. Though it is more commonly found on the wall of the hoof, the sole can also become involved. Clean the hoof well with soap and water and rinse. Put 1/2 teaspoon of tea tree oil into 1/2 cup of water and pour into a spray bottle. Spray the entire hoof and around the coronary band thoroughly once a day. If possible, isolate the pig and keep it in a clean environment until the condition clears.

Foot Rot is a serious condition that affects pigs up to six months of age, especially if they are reared inside on concrete instead of wood floors.

Wounds

Tea tree oil is also very effective on cuts, wounds, bites and stings. Always clean the area thoroughly before treatment. Saturate a cotton ball with tea tree oil and dab directly onto the site. Continue daily until a healthy scab has formed or the bite or sting disappears. The oil will help soothe the pain and aid in healing.

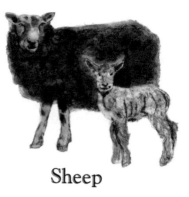

Sheep

Sheep can benefit from tea tree oil in a variety of ways. Skin conditions, minor cuts, abrasions, abscesses and some hoof conditions are treatable with tea tree oil. After shearing, use tea tree oil on any nicks or areas where you may have shaved too closely or burned the skin. Tea tree oil will aid in healing and soothe any burns or irritations. As with treating any animal with a skin condition, it is recommended that you use rubber or latex gloves during treatment.

Skin Conditions

Dermatitis is an inflammation of the skin caused by a variety of agents. Deratophilus Congolensis (or lumpy wool) is a term used when the woolen areas of the body are affected. The term strawberry foot rot is used when the condition affects a portion of the limbs. Isolate the infected animals, then shear away wool to expose affected area. Saturate a cotton ball with tea tree oil and dab directly onto the site. Treat the area 1-2 times per day until the condition has cleared.

Orf

Contagious Ecthyma (Orf) is an infectious dermatitis affecting both sheep and goats. It is encountered in all parts of the world and occurs most commonly in late summer, fall and winter on pasture or feed lots. The lesions develop on the sheep on the lips, as well as in the mouth and occasionally on the feet around the coronet band. Ewes, nursing infected lambs may sometimes develop lesions on the udder. Isolate infected animals until the condition clears. Put 1 drop of tea tree oil onto a cotton swab and dab this onto the lesion of the lips and/or feet 1-2 times per day until scab appears and then falls off. The tea tree oil will aid in healing and help soothe the pain caused from the lesions.

Ringworm

Ringworm is a contagious fungus that affects nearly all animals as well as humans. Though it is uncommon in sheep and goats, when it does occur, the lesions can usually be found on the head, neck and shoulders of the animals. It appears on the skin as a reddish circular lesion causing itching. It is characterized by the sheep rubbing a bare spot and may become more noticeable after shearing.

Clip or shear away any unwanted hair around the site. Wash the area with soap and water and rinse. Pat dry with paper towel and dispose. Saturate a cotton ball with tea tree oil and squeeze out the excess, dab this directly onto the site. Isolate the animal and repeat this treatment 2-3 times per day, until the condition clears. This can be stubborn, so stay with it. Remember with any contagious condition, to disinfect your grooming tools, particularly the shears, to prevent further contamination to other animals.

Sheep Ked

Sheep Ked (sheep tick) is an insect which can spend its entire life on it's host. These ticks can spread rapidly through a flock, especially if they are kept in close quarters. Although shearing removes them, the tick feeds by piercing the skin and sucking blood. They are commonly found on the neck, breast, shoulder, flanks and rump. The ticks cause a defect in the hide called a cockie. This blemish affects the grade and value of the sheep skin. For the best results, treat after shearing. Put 1/2 teaspoon of tea tree oil into 1/2 cup of water, pour this into a spray bottle and spray the animal down thoroughly. The tea tree oil will aid in healing any blemishes and can act as an insect repellent as well.

Sheep Ked, if untreated can blemish the skin and affect the value of the hide, as well as causing discomfort to your animals.

Mange

Sarcoptic mange in sheep, as a rule, occurs usually on the non-woolen skin. Outbreaks, although rare, start on the head and face. Chorioptic mange however, is the most frequent type of mange and is found on the hind legs and between the toes and sometimes on the scrotum of the rams. It is also commonly called leg or foot mange. Itch mite infestation is also common in sheep. To treat these conditions, shear and wash animal with soap and water and rinse. Saturate a cotton ball with tea tree oil and squeeze off the excess. Dab it directly onto the site 2-3 times per day until condition clears. It is best to isolate the animal during treatment.

Photosensitization

Photosensitization occurs world-wide in many species but is most common in cattle and sheep. With lightly pigmented animals, their skin becomes inflamed following long term exposure to ultraviolet rays. It is best to provide shade during treatment and until the condition has cleared. Saturate a cotton ball with tea tree oil and squeeze out the excess. Dab this directly onto the affected area to help soothe the burn and aid in healing.

Sheep Pox

Sheep Pox is a virus that is serious, often fatal and is characterized by wide spread skin eruptions. This condition is confined to parts of southeastern Europe, Africa and Asia. Tea tree oil can help topically by aiding in soothing the pain and irritation of the lesions. Saturate a cotton ball with tea tree oil and dab directly onto the site until the condition clears. A veterinarian should be consulted concerning this condition.

> *Sheep Pox is a virus that is serious, often fatal, and is characterized by wide spread skin eruptions. Consult your veterinarian.*

Warts

Warts are rare in sheep, but if they do occur, they can be transmitted to other sheep but not to other species. Saturate a cotton ball with tea tree oil and squeeze off the excess. Dab directly onto the wart 2-3 times per day until it clears. This treatment can take weeks.

Foot Abscesses

Foot Abscesses develop most often when the soil and pastures are wet. Rams, particularly in their first winter, and ewes during late pregnancy are most affected. The condition may result in lameness and can be caused from foot rot. Remove the animal from the damp environment and provide clean dry housing. Wash the foot thoroughly with soap and water, rinse and dry. Put 1/2 teaspoon of tea tree oil in 1/2 cup of water and pour into a spray bottle. Spray the area thoroughly. Keep the wound clean and allow it to drain. Continue treatment 1-2 times a day until the condition clears.

Foot rot

Foot rot is caused by bacteria and is commonplace in the sheep environment. The condition is also contagious under warm moist conditions. As with foot abscesses, provide a clean dry environment during treatment. Wash the foot thoroughly with soap and water, rinse and dry. Put 1/2 teaspoon of tea tree oil into 1/2 cup of water and pour into a spray bottle. Spray the foot thoroughly. Continue treatment 1-2 times a day until the condition clears.

Wounds

Cuts, wounds, bites and stings can all be treated with tea tree oil. It will aid in healing and soothe any pain or irritation that may accompany the condition. Clean the area thoroughly with soap and water, rinse and pat dry. Saturate a cotton ball with tea tree oil squeezing out any excess, and dab directly onto the site. Repeat 1-2 times a day until the condition clears.

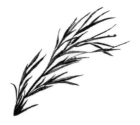

Appendix A

Recommended Reading

Dr. Pitcairn's Complete Guide to Natural
Health for Cats and Dogs
　Richard H. Pitcairn, DVM, PhD &
　Susan Hubble-Pitcairn.
　1995, Rodale Books

Any of the series by Dr. Tim Hawcroft,
BVSc, MACVSc:
A-Z of Horse Diseases and Health Problems
First Aid for Birds
First Aid for Cats
First Aid for Dogs
First Aid for Horses
　Howell Book House, NY.

A-Z of Dog Diseases and Health Problems
　Dick Lane, BScFRAgS, FRCVS and Neil Ewart
　1995, Howell Book House, NY.

The Illustrated Veterinary Guide for Dogs,
Cats, Birds & Exotic Pets
　Chris C. Pinney DVM
　1992, Tab Books - a division of McGraw Hill.

Resources

You can purchase high quality Tea Tree Oil concentrates, extracts, books and products from any of the following companies:

Kali Press (Publisher)
(Books, & products)
PO Box 2169
Pagosa Springs, CO 81147-2169
(970) 264-5200   fax: (970)264-5202
(888) 999-5254(KALI)
email: kalipres@rmi.net

A Natural Path - Cheyanne West (Author)
(Books & products, Alternative Health Magazine for Animals)
PO Box 70
Lewis, CO 81327
(970) 882-8888

Chamisa Ridge
PO Box 23294
Santa Fe NM 87502-3294
(505) 438-4811

Wise Old Nag
PO Box 1140
Ignacio, CO 81137
(970) 808-5563

Derma-E
9400 Lurline Avenue, #C-1
Chatsworth, CA 91311
(800) 521-3342
*Tea tree oil hair and skin care products: shampoo,
conditioner, tea tree oil, vitamin E oil, tea tree oil cream.*

Desert Essence
Ron Gerard, General Manager/Vice President Sales
9510 Vassar Ave., Unit A
Chatsworth, CA 91311
(800) 645-5768   fax: (818) 705-8525
*Tea tree oil health and body care products. Other brand
name: Tea Tree Solutions.*

Essential Care USA, Inc.
Division of Essential Resources, Sydney, Australia
Max Tessler, MD, President
661 Palisade Ave.
Englewood Cliffs, NJ 07632
(201) 567-9004   fax: (201) 567-8853
*Melaleuca oil products. Bulk oil; also retail markets,
health and beauty aids.*

Marco Industries
3431 W. Thunderbird, Suite 144
Phoenix, AZ 85023
(800) 726-1612   (602) 789-7048
email: marco-lesi@juno.com
*Manufactures 100% tea tree oil as a preservative and
antiseptic; antiseptic herbal ointment, soothing cream
in colloidal silver base, suppositories, douche; Convita
tea tree oil toothpaste (New Zealand).*

Thursday Plantation, Inc.
Michael Dean, President
330 Carillo St.
Santa Barbara, CA 93101
(805) 566-0354   fax: (805) 566-9798
Tea tree products.

Trivent Chemical Company
4266 US Rt. One
Monmouth Junction, NJ 08852
Suppliers of raw material to cosmetic/pharmaceutical companies.

Water Jel Technologies
243 Veterans Blvd.
Carlstadt, NJ 07072
Peter D. Cohen, President
(201) 507-8300   fax: (201) 507-8325
Medical supplies, tea tree burn blankets.

Herbs

American Botanical Council
P.O. Box 201660
Austin, TX 78720
(512) 331-8868   fax: (512) 331-1924
email: custserv@herbalgram.org
web site: www.herbalgram.org
Publishes HerbalGram, a quarterly journal geared toward health professionals, industry, and those interested in herb research, market conditions, and regulation. Also provides an Herbal Education Catalog, listing over 300 publications.

Aroma Vera
5901 Rodeo Rd.
Los Angeles, CA 90016-4312
(800) 669-9514   fax: (310) 280-0395

Aura Cacia
101 Paymaster Rd.
Weaverville, CA 96093
(800) 437-3301   fax: (800) 717-4372

Herb Pharm
20260 Williams Highway
Williams, OR 97544
(800) 348-4372   fax: (541) 846-6112

Herb Research Foundation
1007 Pearl Street, Ste. 200
Boulder, CO 80302
(303) 449-2265   fax: (303) 449-7849
Botanical research services. Co-publishes HerbalGram.

Starwest Botanicals, Inc.
11253 Trade Center Dr.
Rancho Cordova, CA 95742
(916) 638-8100
(800) 800-4372   fax:(916) 638-8293
Tea tree oil to wholesale customers only.

Multi-Level Companies

Melaleuca Inc.
3910 S. Yellowstone Hwy.
Idaho Falls, ID 83402
(208) 522-0700   fax: (208) 528-2090

Espial USA Ltd.
7045 South Fulton Street, Ste. 200
Englewood, CO 80112
(800) 695-5555   fax: (303) 792-3933
Personal care products containing tea tree oil.

Canada

Australian Bodycare of Canada, Ltd.
Vancouver, BC
Canada
(604) 922-2562   fax: (604) 922-2576
email: abc_ca@istar.ca
web site: www.beautynet.com/abc
Direct importer of tea tree oil, manufacturer and distributor of the Professional Therapeutic Tea Tree Oil range of products.

Brueckner Group
Ron Jean
4717 14th Avenue
Markham, Ontario, L3S 3k3
Canada
(905) 479-2121   fax: (905) 479-2122
Manufactures tea tree oil skin care products.

PET RESOURCES

World Wide Pet Supply Association
Mr. Douglas Poindexter- Exec. Vice Pres.
406 S. First Ave.
Arcadia, CA 91006-3829
(626) 447-2222   fax (626) 447-8350
e-mail: info@wwpsa.com
website: www.wwpsa.om
Foods, products, services - USA oldest Assoc.

Pet Industry Distributors Association
5024-R Campbell Blvd.
Baltimore, MD 21236-5974
(410) 931-8100   fax (410) 931-8111
e-mail: sking@unidial.com
website: www.pida.org
Booklet available listing hundreds of pet store distributors

Pet Sitters International
Ms. Patti Moran, President
418 E. King St.
King, NC 27021
(336) 983-9222   fax (336) 983-3755
e-mail: petsittin@aols.net
website: www.petsit.com
Newsletter, info line, convention,
Professional Pet Sitters list.: (800)268-7487

Pet Age Magazine
Karen Long-MacLeod, Editor
200 S. Michigan Ave. #840
Chicago, IL 60604

(312) 663-4040   fax (312) 663-5676
e-mail: petage@aol.com
25,000 subjects, publishing, grooming & board.

Pet Food Express
Mr. Mark Witroil - Buyer
701 Whitney St.
San Leandro, CA 94577
(510) 567-9999
Books on pet care

The Pet Dealer
Mr. Mark Hawver, Exec. Editor
Cygnus Publishing
445 Broad Hollow Rd.
Melville, NY 11747
(516) 845-2700 fax (516) 845-2797
(800) 547-7377 circulation/ads/subscription
Publications to 11,000 retail stores.

Pets Plus Animal Kingdom
206 W. Burlington
Fairfield, IA 52556
(515) 472-6971

Natural Pet Magazine
Ms. Lisa A. Hanks - Editor
PO Box 6050
Mission Viejo, CA 92690
Magazine on Holistic care for your best friends

Pet Life Magazine
Ms. Jana Murphy, Managing Editor
Magnolia Media Group
2 Tandy Center, suite 1400
300 W. 3rd St.
Fort Worth, TX 76102
(817) 921-9201
Your companion animal magazine

Steppin' Out
P.O. Box 1196
Spring Hill, TN 37174-1196
(615) 274-2261   fax:(615) 274-2529
e-mail: paddy@edge.net
Show horse & dressage publication

Alternative Approaches to Pet Care

A Natural Path
Ms. Cheyanne West
PO Box 70
Lewis, CO 81327
(970) 882-8888   fax: (970) 882-8888
ANPRRDLCW@webtv.net
website: www.inergy.com/anaturalpath
Homeopathy, supplements, newsletter on animal health care

Alternative Medical Approach to Animals
Marie Cheralu-Williams, DVM
(303) 443-0202 - *for consultations* fax: (303) 494-4004
e-mail: mcw@boulder.earthnet.net

Academy of Veterinary Homeopathy (AHV)
751 NE 168th St.
North Miami, FL 33162-2427
(305) 652-5372   fax: (305) 653-7244
email: avh@naturalholistic.com
        academy@docb.com
can refer you to a trained homeopathic veterinarian

American Holistic Veterinary Medical Association (AHVMA)
2214 Old Emmorton Rd.
Bel Air, MD 21014
(410) 569-0795   fax: (410) 569-2346
email: AHVMA@compuserve.com
referrals, membership, information, and directory

American Veterinary Chiropractic Association (AVCA)
623 Main
Hillsdale, IL 61257
(309) 658-2920   fax: (309) 658-2622

International Veterinary Acupuncture Society (IVAS)
P.O. Box 1478
Longmont, CO 80502
(303) 682-1167   fax: (303) 682-1168
email: IVASOffice@aol.com
information, membership and directory

On World Wide Web
Information, referrals, articles

http://www.AltVetMed.com

http://www.holisticvet.com/core.html

http://www.designexperts.com/wholisticvet/

http://www.acmepet.com/canine/market/k9
first aid for cats and dogs

http://www.petsynergy.com
how to find holistic consultations

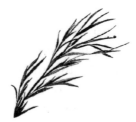

Appendix B

TEA TREE INFORMATION
& SPECIFICATIONS

TEA TREE OIL*
Melaleuca alternifolia: common name "tea tree". A member of the laurel tree family, unusual variety indigenous to the east coast of New South Wales, Australia. Natural stands of trees usually found in low lying, swampy areas. Trees produced from seed are now being grown on plantations in the region. Seeds are quite small, and the quality of the seed affects the output of the plantation. Seedlings take seven to ten days to germinate in the summer months; when ten to fifteen cm. tall, they are transplanted.

Essential Oil: steam-distilled essence from the root, bark, flower, and/or leaf of plants. Many oils are used in healing, aromatherapy, and culinary uses.
* excerpted from Australian Tea Tree Oil Guide, Kali Press, 1997.

Composition of Tea Tree Essential Oil: Naturally-occurring essential oil, colorless or pale yellow. If discolorations appear, it usually indicates an inferior distillation process. Impurities and weeds in the distillation process may also affect the color. The oil is distilled from leaves of Melaleuca alternifolia, consisting chiefly of terpinenes, cymenes, pinenes, terpineols, cineole, sesquiterpenes, and sequiterpene alcohols. Pleasant characteristic odor with a terebinthinate taste. If odor is strong and varies from batch to batch, it may indicate impurities at the time of distillation.

Action: Pure tea Tree Oil conforming to Australian standard A. S. D. 175, revised 1985 (AS 2782-1985) and 1996 (ISO 4730) is a powerful broad-range antiseptic, fungicide, and bactericide. The main component is terpinen-4-ol (T-4-ol). Optimal activity at 35-40% w/v. Its bacterial action is increased in the presence of blood, serum, pus and necrotic tissue. It is able to penetrate deeply into infected tissue and pus, mix with these, and cause them to slough off while leaving a healthy surface. The oil has a very low toxicity, and is virtually a non-irritant even to sensitive tissues. Because of its lower cineole level, tea tree oil is less toxic and less irritating than eucalyptus oil. Be aware that some unknown eucalyptus oils have been blended with a synthetic form of terpinen-4-o, which alters the chemical composition.

Indications: (Different species are effected by different varieties of diseases with similar common names, see specific sub-chapters for individual uses with specific animals.) Cuts, scratches, abrasions, burns, sunburn, prickly heat, insect bites and stings, scalds, allergic and itching dermatoses, lice, mites, ear mites, warts, ringworm, eczema, mange and scabies (different animals are especially suseptible to different kinds of mange - see each one specifically), pox viruses, thrush, quittor, greasy heel, foot rot, Candida albicans, Pityriasis Rosa, Contagious Ecthyma, Sheep Ked.

Precautions: Pure oil will dissolve certain plastics. Store only in glass (preferably amber) containers in a cool place. Bulk tea tree oil holds up much better from damage, deterioration, and oxidation if initially stored and shipped in steel drums.

Extremely sensitive skin may need dilution of the pure oil. Dilution of 1:250 are still bacteriostatic against pathogenic streptococci and staphylococci, typhous, pneumococcus, and gonococcus.

WEIGHTS AND MEASURES/CONVERSION TABLE

(Australian common usage to U. S. common usage)

1 milliliter (ml)	= 0.0338/fl. ounce
10 milliliter	= 0.338/fl. ounce
1 kilogram (kg)	= 2.2046 pounds

Recommendations & Precautions

Avoid any contact of tea tree oil with the eyes.

Do not drink tea tree oil.

Keep out of reach of children.

Do not use or store full strength tea tree oil in plastic containers.

Do not use or store tea tree oil around homeopathic remedies, as it will contaminate your remedy. Keep cap on tight and store in a cool, dry place.

Never put tea tree oil full strength directly into an animals ear, as it may burn the delicate skin; dilute it or put on cotton swab, being careful to squeeze out any excess.

When you need to mix tea tree oil with other oil, we recommend a non-fragrant oil such as vitamin E or even a sunflower seed oil.

When treating any contagious skin conditions, wear protective gloves. It is always best to disinfect the tools you use (e.g., scissors etc.) and / or dispose of any paper towels, cotton balls etc. Do not reuse the towels until they too have been disinfected and washed. It is best to disinfect their cages each time you treat the animal so as not to reinfect them.

When removing ticks, always use gloves or at least keep a barrier between your skin and the tick, Tick Fever and Lyme's Disease have been transmitted by touching infected ticks.

INDEX

A

abscesses 5,11,18,19,37, 62,70, 73, 76, 80, 88, 90, 99, 100, 101, 105, 123

abrasions 20, 37, 47,61, 123

alfalfa 103

B

bacteria 39, 53, 123

barbering 36

bedding 25

birds 31-35

blankets 53, 65

brushes 65, 80

buckets 63

C

cages 25, 31, 32, 33, 35, 37, 38, 39, 40, 45

Candida Albicans 102, 123

Canine Distemper, 44

carbolic acid 77, 80

cats 9-23

cattle 95-101

Chorioptic Mange 91, 97, 109

Cow Pox 98

cross-firing wounds 77

D

Demodectic Mange 16, 90

dental problems 22

Deratophilus Congolensis 106

dermatitis 5, 37, 39, 41, 62, 63, 79, 106, 107, 123

disinfect 11, 12, 14, 24, 25, 31, 33, 39, 40, 47, 53, 61, 62, 66, 74, 80, 85, 96, 98, 103, 108

E

ear mites 13, 39, 42, 44, 45

eczema 46, 87, 123

F

farm uses 79

feather picking 32

Feline Leukemia Virus 44

ferrets 44-45

fleas 5, 16, 17, 18, 36, 39, 40, 41, 44, 45, 55

foot abscesses 110

foot rot 93, 104

fungus 5, 11, 63, 79, 91, 96, 102, 123

G

galls 71

gangrene 86

general liniments 73

gerbils 31, 37-38

Gingivitis 87

Goat Pox 87,92, 99

goats 86-95

Greasy Heel 73, 78
Greasy Pig Disease 47
grooming tools 25, 63, 80, 97
guinea pigs 31, 35-37

H

hair loss 36, 40, 42, 44
hamsters 31, 37, 38
hand cream 1, 53
heartworm 44
hives 21, 73
hoof conditions 73, 93, 100,104
homeopathic remedies 131,132
horses 59-81
hot spots, 17
household uses,

I

insect bites 21, 47, 61, 73, 99
insect repellents 11, 21, 55, 56, 77
intestinal parasites 45, 47
isopropyl alcohol, 55

L

lacerations 32, 61, 99
leg mange, 74, 91
lice, 15, 16, 64, 123
lesions, 37, 64, 86, 97
liniments, 5, 61, 73
lip balm, 53
lumpy wool, 106
lyme disease, 67

M

mange 16, 36, 37, 39, 40, 47, 65, 66, 87, 88, 96, 97, 109, 123
massage oil 55
Melaleuca Alternifolia, 6, 122, 123
miniature pot-bellied pigs 31, 46-47
mites 15,16, 31, 36, 45, 53, 65, 89, 90, 91, 97, 123
mouth abscesses 21

O

oils 55
Orf 107
over-reaching wounds 77

P

Papillomas 32
papule 92, 99, 103
parasites 36, 37, 44, 45
petroleum jelly, 51, 53, 70
photosensitization 88, 95, 96, 103, 109
pigs 101-105
Pityriasis Rosa 103, 123
Pneumococcus 123
Pododermatitis 35
pot-bellied pigs 31, 46-47
Pox Virus 43, 123
precautions 132
pregnancy 35, 110
pressure sores 71
Psoroptic Mange 89, 90, 97
punctures 18, 31, 32

Pustular
Psoriaform Dermatitis 103

Q
Quittor 73, 77, 123

R
rabbits 39-44
rashes 21, 61
referrals 123, 124
ringworm 14, 16, 36, 39, 40, 63, 87, 96, 102, 107, 123

S
saddle sores 71
Saheep Ked (sheep tick) 108, 123
salves 5, 11, 46, 51, 61, 62, 63, 87, 91, 96, 102, 107, 123
Sarcoptic Mange 16, 65, 89, 90, 97, 107, 109
Scabies 65, 89, 123
Seborrhea 46
Seedy Toes, 94, 96
seizures 36
Septicaemia 104
shampoos, 5, 11, 25, 54, 56, 61
sheath cleaners 68
sheep 106-111
Sheep Scab 90
Sheep Pox 110
skin conditions 12, 35, 39, 54, 61, 85, 86, 87, 95, 96, 101, 104
Sore Hocks 39
Staphylococci 89, 123
St. John's Wort 88, 96, 103

Strawberry Foot Rot 106
Streptococci 89, 123
Summer Sores 61
sunburn 13, 46, 69, 87, 88, 95, 96, 103, 123

T
tea tree oil, history 123
teats 92, 93, 95, 99
ticks 5, 16, 36, 40, 41, 55, 66, 67, 123
thrush 75, 123
Typhous 123

U
udders 92, 95, 107
ulcers 21, 35, 39, 46, 70

W
warts 5, 13, 43
wounds 18, 20, 32, 33, 47, 61, 70, 99

V
vaccination sites 61
vaseline 51, 53, 62, 70
Vesticular Stomatitis 61
Vitamin E 13, 26, 69, 70, 73

Y
yeast infections 5

About the Author

$\mathcal{C}$ heyanne West is a Homeopathic consultant and educator who specializes in working with animals. She is the author of numerous articles on treating horses and other animals with homeopathy as well as other alternative therapies. For the past 20 years she has owned, trained and shown both horses and dogs. She operates an after-care service for horses which offers post-operative care, general injury care and maintenance, as well as foaling. She also takes horses in training for behavioral and physical therapy.

Her training in homeopathy began many years ago with her introduction to Dr. Robin Murphy, ND. PHD., the Director of The Hahnemann Academy of North America (HANA). Since 1995 Cheyanne has since pursued her own research in homeopathy, concentrating on the treatment of animals.

From 1984 to present, she has worked with the Colorado Division of Wildlife and the Southern Ute Indian Tribe as a wildlife/hunter education instructor. There she assisted in numerous wildlife relocation projects, aerial game counts, as well as wildlife management. She is a former Vet Tech and has many years experience in alternative therapies for animals as well as animal health care.

Cheyanne established "A Natural Path" in 1995, which offers a complete mail order catalog on alternative medicines, books, and tapes, as well as a variety of homeopathic emergency remedy kits which she designed specifically for cats, dogs, horses, caged birds, wildlife, cattle, sheep, goats and pigs. She offers day long and weekend workshops on alternative medicine, homeopathy and animal health care. Most recently, she has developed a newsletter called *"Alternatives - A Natural Path to Animal Health Care"*. Published four times a year, this newsletter is packed with articles and helpful tips on choosing and using alternative therapies for animals.

Throughout all of her work and research, Cheyanne is committed to providing accurate information on alternative health care for animals in a most direct and simple manner. Those who have attended her workshops appreciate her common sense — no nonsense way of communicating.

Currently Cheyanne lives and writes in the Four Corners area of Colorado. She is a contributing writer to *Australian Tea Tree Oil Guide - 3rd Edition* and currently offers *Australian Tea Tree Oil: First Aid for Animals,* published by Kali Press, Pagosa Springs, CO. Her next book due out in September is entitled *A Natural Path for Horses* - Homeopathy and Other Alternative Therapies published by A Natural Path, PO Box 70, Lewis, CO 81327

Do you have any success stories using tea tree oil with animals? Tell us about it!

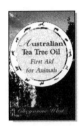
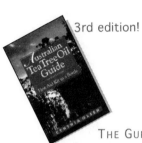

KALI SIDELINES

BIRTHING THE BABES OF THE LIGHT

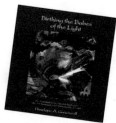

A new book about conscious sacred birthing and the unusual children being born today....for parents, grandparents, teachers, midwives, nurses, and anyone involved with birthing, children, and co-creative endeavors.
by Penelope Greenwell
ISBN 0-9648147-8-1 $17.00*

HIGH QUALITY, PURE TEA TREE OIL

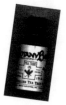

-pharmaceutical grade of Tea Tree Oil in one ounce bottles- contains over 35% Terpinen & less than 5% Cineole
1 oz Botany Bay Tea Tree Oil $9.95*

ESSIAC FORMULA IN TINCTURE FORM!!

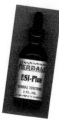

10-15 drops makes one cup of tea....
The Ojibwa Formula renowned for its effectiveness against conditions including Cancer, Aids, & Diabetes, also a powerful Liver and Colon detoxifying flush...
2 oz Herbals Essiac Tincture $29.95*

Kali Press
P.O. Box 2169
Pagosa Springs, Colorado 81147
970-264-5200 fax: 970-264-5202
e-mail: kalipres@rmi.net
Order Line: 888-999-5254 (KALI)

Shipping and handling not included. Please call for prices.
wholesale and distributor inquiries welcomed !